Alcohol and Sexuality:

An Annotated Bibliography on Alcohol Use, Alcoholism, and Human Sexual Behavior

Alcohol and Sexuality:

An Annotated Bibliography on Alcohol Use, Alcoholism, and Human Sexual Behavior

by Timothy J. O'Farrell, Ph.D.
and Carolyn A. Weyand, Ph.D.
with Diane Logan, Ph.D.

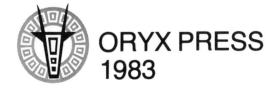

ORYX PRESS
1983

The rare Arabian Oryx is believed to have inspired the myth of the unicorn. This desert antelope became virtually extinct in the early 1960s. At that time several groups of international conservationists arranged to have 9 animals sent to the Phoenix Zoo to be the nucleus of a captive breeding herd. Today the Oryx population is over 400 and herds have been returned to reserves in Israel, Jordan, and Oman.

Library of Congress Cataloging in Publication Data

O'Farrell, Timothy J.
    Alcohol and sexuality.

    Includes index.
    1. Alcoholics—Sexual behavior—Abstracts.
I. Weyand, Carolyn A. II. Logan, Diane. III. Title.
[DNLM: 1. Alcohol drinking—Abstracts. 2. Alcoholism
—Abstracts. 3. Sex behavior—Drug effects—Abstracts.
4. Sex disorders—Chemically induced—Abstracts.
ZWM 274 031a]
HV5201.S48033   1983   016.6166'9   82-73732
ISBN 0-89774-040-8

If a great thing can be done at all,
it can be done easily. But it is that
kind of ease with which a tree
blossoms after long years of gathering strength.

John Ruskin
The Author's Kalendar, 1920

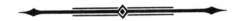

Dedicated to:

My mother and father,
Helen & Robert O'Farrell
TOF

My husband,
Theodore G. Weyand
CAW

Table of Contents

Preface

A close connection between alcohol use and sexual behavior has been documented in most cultures since the beginning of written history. In literature, the often quoted speech of the porter in Shakespeare's *MacBeth* summarizes what many of us, scientists and laypersons alike, have discovered about sex and alcohol: "drink . . . provoketh the desire but taketh away the performance." Paradoxically, beliefs to the contrary have persisted through history, and sex and alcohol remain closely allied in the beliefs and behavior of many individuals and cultures today.

With the advent of the sexual revolution in the past decade, we have seen a dramatic increase in the number of titles on sex and alcohol in the scientific and clinical literature. Laboratory studies of alcohol's effect on the psychological and physiological aspects of human sexual response have appeared in growing numbers. Masters and Johnson reported alcohol use or abuse to be the second most frequent cause of secondary erectile dysfunction. A number of publications and conferences have urged open discussion of alcoholics' sexual problems, education of alcoholism professionals and paraprofessionals in sexuality, and application of newly developed sex counseling and therapy techniques to the alcoholic population.

Despite the recent interest in the sexual adjustment problems of alcoholics and in the effects of alcohol on normal human sexuality, it is difficult for the interested reader to find publications on this topic. The existing literature on alcohol and human sexuality is widely scattered throughout clinical and research journals and not readily available in any convenient place. This means that even sophisticated researchers are not aware of highly relevant work outside their immediate areas of investigation. Clinicians writing to educate their professional peers or their alcoholic patients frequently show ignorance of many relevant scientific studies.

Purpose of the Bibliography

Preparation of this annotated bibliography was undertaken in recognition of the increasing interest in sexuality and alcohol use and abuse and in response to the current need for a comprehensive and extensive reference resource in the field. Physicians, psychiatrists, psychologists, nurses, social workers, counselors, and others involved in research, education, or treatment in the sexuality and alcoholism fields will find this a valuable resource. Those designing alcohol education and sex education programs will find this a valuable compendium of primary source materials on which to base their efforts. This bibliography has been developed to serve the need for ready access to research and clinical work conducted in this field and to aid in locating sources of additional information. We hope that readers will turn to these original sources when needed and that our annotations will help them to decide on the nature and direction of further reading to expand their knowledge.

Scope and Organization

This annotated bibliography on alcohol and human sexuality brings together materials on alcohol and sex published from 1900 to 1982 for easy access by researchers, clinicians, and educators. Materials included focus on the aspects of sexuality concerning sexual arousal, orgasm, and attitudes about sexual behavior; material on sex roles, sex differences, and reproduction have been excluded.

The first chapter deals with alcohol's short-term effects on sexual behavior and the biological underpinnings of sexual behavior in social drinkers and alcoholics, the long-term effects of chronic alcohol abuse on the endocrine functioning necessary for sexual activity, and the aphrodisiac properties attributed to alcohol. The second chapter explores sexual dysfunction and sexual adjustment of male and female alcoholics. One section presents information on the nature of problems reported by alcoholics; another addresses sex therapy and education. The third chapter focuses on the social and cultural issues surrounding sexual behaviors as related to alcohol and alcoholism. The concluding chapter presents broad-based literature reviews, position papers, and commentary. Each chapter begins with a detailed description of its contents and informs the reader about how the citations are organized within the chapter.

Acknowledgements

A donation to Harvard University for the first author's research from Ayerst Laboratories, makers of the drug Antabuse which is used in alcoholism treatment, was essential to the completion of this bibliography and is gratefully acknowledged. We are grateful to the Rutgers University Center for Alcohol Studies (RUCAS) and the National Clearinghouse for Alcohol Information (NCALI) for permission to reproduce abstracts of materials cited in the computerized abstracting systems maintained by these organizations. The abbreviated designation for the appropriate organization is placed at the end of each abstract to indicate the source from which the abstract was taken. Additional abstracts, taken from the author's summary accompanying the publication—designated by ''(Author)'' after the abstract—are reproduced by permission of the publisher of the article. Abstracts that are followed by no source designation were prepared by the authors of this bibliography.

A special thank you goes to Dr. Diane Logan, whose assistance with the completion of this bibliography brought our efforts to a timely end.

Timothy J. O'Farrell
Harvard Medical School
Boston, Massachusetts
Carolyn A. Weyand
University of Connecticut
Storrs, Connecticut

The Search: Method and Sources

The search for the publications annotated in this bibliography made use of a variety of resources. Computerized database searches launched our efforts. As titles became known to us, we obtained copies of each publication. The contents of each was reviewed for its relevance to alcohol and sexual behavior, and the accompanying reference list was closely scanned for more titles. Searches through journals on alcoholism or sexuality produced additional titles. Unpublished bibliographies from a variety of specialized organizations helped to fill out our growing list of titles.

Computerized Database Searches

Citation lists were obtained through the computerized retrieval services of the National Library of Medicine and through computerized searches of *Psychological Abstracts* and *Index Medicus*. The National Clearinghouse for Alcohol Information of the National Institute on Alcohol Abuse and Alcoholism and the Information Services Division of the Center of Alcohol Studies at Rutgers University also supplied computerized searches.

Existing Bibliographies

We discovered a number of unpublished bibliographies in our search. They often lacked annotations and were of limited scope, yet they were helpful in opening search avenues. The Kinsey Institute for Sex Research at Indiana University has several specialized bibliographies—e.g., *Drugs and Sex Behavior, Alcohol and Sex Behavior, Alcoholism & Homosexuality*—which catalog the relevant items in their collection. The Information Services Division of the Rutgers Center of Alcohol Studies publishes the bibliography *Recent Topics in Alcohol Studies: Sexuality (#A680)*. This bibliography is partially annotated and contains representative, current publications. The National Council on Alcoholism and the Wisconsin Clearinghouse supplied lists of material on homosexuality and alcoholism. Complete addresses for these and other sources of material can be found in the appendices. The present bibliography also cites and includes relevant titles from other, previously published bibliographies.

Other Sources of Titles

Despite the convenience of existing bibliographies and computerized databases, much of the search consisted of painstaking review of an assortment of publications: past volumes of major alcoholism journals and sex research/therapy journals, tables of contents from sexology periodicals for laypersons and professionals, announcements of symposia and workshops devoted to alcoholism or sexuality, advertisements for books on sexuality or alcohol, and reference lists from relevant journal articles and book chapters. The *Journal of Studies on Alcohol* proved to be particularly helpful. In addition to being a source of original publications, every other issue contains abstracts of books and articles published elsewhere in the alcoholism field.

Compiling and Annotating

As we obtained copies of each of the publications cited, they were reviewed for their suitability for inclusion. In general, any publication providing information on human sexual behavior and alcohol use was included, even when the primary thrust of the publication was only tangentially related. For example, articles dealing primarily with sex-role conflict in women alcoholics were included when they addressed sexual behavior in the context of sex roles. Once included, articles were then categorized by content for chapter placement. Category descriptions can be found at the beginning of each chapter.

In annotating each citation, we made use of existing abstracts whenever possible. Our primary sources for existing abstracts were: (1) the Classified Abstract Archive of the Alcohol Literature located at the Rutgers University Center of Alcohol Studies (RUCAS), (2) the computerized database of the National Clearinghouse for Alcohol Information (NCALI), and (3) the author's abstract or summary accompanying the publication. Abstracts taken from one of these 3 sources are used with permission, and each is indicated by a parenthetical designation appearing at the end of the abstract. (To maintain consistency, minor changes have been made in some of the annotations.)

For about 50% of our entries, suitable abstracts did not exist, so abstracts were written to provide the reader with the aspect of alcohol and sexuality addressed in the publication and a brief synopsis of the relevant content.

The reader will find occasional unannotated citations of foreign language publications. These are citations of relevant foreign publications for which no English translation or summary exists. Many foreign language publications provide English summaries, and these have been reproduced when available. Translations were sought for those items without English summaries. Unfortunately, prohibitive costs of translation services severely limited our efforts to a few recent publications. For the sake of completeness, the untranslated publications were cited, albeit without annotation, with the hope of their usefulness to some readers.

I. Effects of Alcohol Use and Abuse on Sexual Function

Introduction
A. Effects of Alcohol on Sexual Behavior
    1. Both Sexes (or Gender Unspecified)
    2. Females
    3. Males
    4. Alcohol as an Aphrodisiac

B. Effects of Alcohol on Sex Hormones
    1. Individuals without Cirrhosis
        a. Females
        b. Males
    2. Alcoholic Cirrhosis and Sexual Behavior
        a. Both Sexes
        b. Females
        c. Males

Introduction

This first chapter contains explorations of the ways alcohol influences sexual behavior. Many of the publications are data-based research reports providing information on both alcoholics and social drinkers. Two sections divide this chapter according to the pathway of influence being addressed—(A) psychological and social and (B) physiological. Section A addresses the cultural and psychological means whereby alcohol influences sexual behavior. Here, the reader will find sociological surveys, reports of controlled laboratory studies, and commentary on alcohol's ability to enhance or diminish the sexual experience. The material in this chapter treats the role of alcohol within the sexual situation and not the long-range consequences of chronic alcohol abuse on sexual adjustment (which is covered in Chapter II). For example, the entries in this chapter include: studies comparing sexual fantasy and imagery produced by college students who have consumed alcohol with that produced by subjects receiving no alcohol; laboratory studies of differences in sexual arousal and orgasm as a function of alcohol dosage, situational variables, and expectancies; and sociological surveys of college students or businesspersons about their drinking and sexual activities.

For the reader's convenience, the titles in Section A are grouped into 4 subsections. The items in the first contain information concerning the effects of alcohol on the sexual experiences of both men and women. Some of these report on studies using both males and females; others do not specify gender, and their contents can be applied to both sexes. The second and third subsections group titles into those dealing with effects specific to females and those specific to males, respectively. The last subsection presents publications containing information on the aphrodisiac properties of alcohol. Many of the items give current opinions about alcohol as an aphrodisiac; others present information about alcohol as an aphrodisiac from a historical perspective.

The contents of Section B focus on the endocrine system as the pathway through which alcohol affects sexual behavior. The publications presented here report findings from studies examining the effect of alcohol on hormone metabolism and hormone homeostasis as determinants of sexual interest, arousal, and orgasm in humans. The first subsection concerns hormone metabolism among social drinkers and alcoholics without detectable liver damage. The titles are grouped by gender of the persons studied with publications on females appearing first. The second subsection has material on the endocrine functioning of alcoholics with cirrhosis of the liver. In these publications, the disturbed sex hormone metabolism of the liver-damaged alcoholic is studied and discussed, focusing on the implications for sexual functioning. Among the entries are review and theory papers, reports of empirical research, and recommendations to physicians who are called upon to treat sexual problems in patients with cirrhosis. Again, for the reader's convenience, entries begin with the group of titles that do not specify gender or that include both. These are followed by entries on females only, which, in turn, are followed by those on males only.

Unfortunately, the research on alcohol and sex hormones in women has concentrated on child-bearing and the menstrual cycle. Efforts to locate relevant studies revealed a striking paucity of material on female sexual behavior, which is reflected in the sparseness of this group of entries.

A. Effects of Alcohol on Sexual Behavior

1. Both Sexes (or Gender Unspecified)

1. Athanasiou, R., Shaver, P., & Tavris, C. Sex. *Psychology Today*, 1970, *4*, 37–44.

More than 20,000 readers of *Psychology Today* responded to a questionnaire on sexuality. A portion of the questionnaire was devoted to alcohol and marijuana use. Tabulation of responses on alcohol effects on intercourse is as follows: enhances enjoyment—males 45%, females 68%; no effect—males 13%, females 11%; decreases enjoyment—males 42%, females 21%. A number of respondents qualified their answers to indicate that consuming large amounts of alcohol had an adverse effect on enjoyment. Broken down by religious preference: enhances enjoyment—61% of the Unitarians, Protestants, and Catholics, 53% of the Atheists, and 51% of the Jews; no effect—Atheists and Catholics 11%, Jews 12%, Unitarians 14%, Protestants 27%, and Catholics 28%. The effects of alcohol are more diverse than effects of marijuana.

2. Bowker, L. H. The relationship between sex, drugs, and sexual behavior on a college campus. *Drug Forum*, 1978, *7*, 69–80.

Questionnaires on drug use, source of drug supply, and dating behavior were answered by 520 college students; 92% reported ever using alcohol, 65% marijuana, and 26% other recreational drugs. Men were supplied by other men in nearly 90% of the cases for all drugs combined; women commonly received alcohol from other women in 38% of the cases, but all drugs combined were mostly supplied by men (often without monetary remuneration). A higher proportion of independent women than sorority sisters received all of their alcohol, marijuana, and other drugs from men. In many cases women had sexual relations with their drug suppliers. Most men said they had used drugs at least once to make their partners more sexually willing or responsive; 70% of the drinkers (64% of the total sample) reported being involved in a seduction using alcohol; 42% of the men and 45% of the women reported being seduced at least once with either alcohol, marijuana, or other drugs. A majority of respondents saw all 3 drug categories as increasing the incidence of sexual behavior at least some of the time; 17% of men and women reported that marijuana and 27% that alcohol often or always increased the incidence of sexual behavior; 46% reported that alcohol sometimes and 27% that it rarely or never increased the incidence of sexual behavior. Only 15% of the men and 13% of the women said alcohol increased their sexual enjoyment, compared with 26% and 24%, respectively, for marijuana. The results indicate that college men have added alcohol and other drugs to their repertoire of interpersonal mechanisms for the control of relationships with women. (RUCAS)

3. Brown, S. A., Goldman, M. S., Inn, A., & Anderson, L. R. Expectations of reinforcement from alcohol: Their domain and relation to drinking patterns. *Journal of Consulting and Clinical Psychology*, 1980, *48*, 419–426.

Since previous research has suggested that some behavioral effects of alcohol are due to expectancies (i.e., expected rather than actual psychopharmacological effects of alcohol), the domain of alcohol reinforcement expectancies was investigated. A questionnaire was developed from interviews with 125 men and women from the Detroit metropolitan area who had widely diversified drinking patterns and was refined statistically using responses from an additional 400 subjects (44% women). The refined version was administered to 440 nonalcoholics and a factor analysis was performed. The 6 independent belief factors extracted were that alcohol (1) transforms experiences in a positive way, (2) enhances social and physical pleasures, (3) enhances sexual performance and experience, (4) increases power and aggression, (5) increases social assertiveness, and (6) reduces tensions. Canonical variate analysis clarified relationships between these factors and the subjects' customary alcohol use and demographic variables. The more global factors were related to light consumption, while an increased expectation of sexual and aggressive behavior was characteristic for subjects drinking more heavily. The theoretical and practical implications of these findings are discussed. (RUCAS)

4. Gaupp. Alkohol und geschlechtsleben. [Alcohol and sex life.] *Zentralblatt für die gesamte Neurologie und Psychiatrie*, 1923, *32*, 3.

Remarks on the effect of alcohol on sex life. Alcohol strengthens the sex drive and lowers control over it. This peculiar effect distinguishes it from all other intoxicants.

5. Hoffman, J. *Here's to your health: The sobering facts about social drinking.* Emmaus, PA: Rodale, 1980.

This book is intended for average social drinkers who want to know the effects of their own individual drinking patterns on their total health and behavior. Documented charts and tables are presented. The effects of drinking on the heart, brain, and other internal organs and on human performance, personality, and sexuality as well as the effects of alcohol on adolescents and pregnant women are considered. Alcohol and its relation to nutrition and cancer are included along with a list of widely used drugs that may interact badly with alcohol. The last chapter contains ways to avoid drinking in social situations. (RUCAS)

6. Lang, A. R. *Drinking and disinhibition: Contributions from psychological research.* Paper presented at the Conference on Alcohol and Disinhibition, Berkeley, CA, February 1981.

Some contributions from psychology to a comprehensive theory of drinking and disinhibition are outlined. Ways of determining whether or not alcohol per se is causally related to the behavior of drinkers are discussed. Studies employing a "balanced placebo" design, which permits both separate and interactive examination of psychological and pharmacological effects of drinking on behavior, are reviewed. While emphasis is given to disinhibited expression of aggressive, sexual, and other behavior with direct and important social implications, an account of the effects of drinking on other behaviors is also provided. Also addressed is the question of determining how certain nonpathological individual differences (gender and drinking experiences) might influence both beliefs about drinking and its actual effects. An effort at integrating the findings of psychological research into the broad theories of drinking and disinhibition is attempted. (NCALI)

7. Lolli, G. The taboo on tenderness. In G. Lolli, *Social drinking: The effects of alcohol.* New York: Collier Books, 1961.

Repression of tender feelings resulting from the internalization of taboos on tenderness leads to coldness and aloofness with loved ones. This pattern has been demonstrated by men and women in our society. It can interfere with parent-child relationships and with the sexual relationship between spouses. Sexual difficulties may be due not to specific sexual inhibitions but to shame connected with expression of warmth and tender feelings. Alcohol may temporarily dissolve the taboo, allowing the individual to engage in exchanges of tenderness. Use of alcohol is an unhealthy solution, which at extremes can produce a distorted or explosive release of inhibition. Recognizing and overcoming the taboo is required for healthy satisfaction in intimate relationships.

8. Marlatt, G. A., & Rohsenow, D. J. Think-drink effect. *Psychology Today,* December 1981, pp. 60–69; 93.

To investigate how cognitive processes influence reaction to alcohol (the "think-drink" effect), a study was conducted using a balanced-placebo design. Thirty-two social drinkers and 32 alcoholics were divided into the 4 conditions of the balanced-placebo method: (1) expect alcohol/receive alcohol, (2) expect alcohol/receive no alcohol, (3) expect no alcohol/receive alcohol, and (4) expect no alcohol/receive no alcohol. Subjects in the 2 "expect alcohol" groups believed they would be comparing brands of vodka, while those in the 2 "expect no alcohol" groups were told they would be comparing brands of tonic water. Half the subjects in the

"expect alcohol" condition and half of those in the "expect no alcohol" condition received vodka and tonic; the rest of the subjects were given tonic water. Results showed that expectancy was the main influence on the total amount consumed by both social drinkers and alcoholics. Findings from other studies using the balanced-placebo design are reported and indicate that people's beliefs about drinking are linked with some drinkers' aggressive behavior. Findings on the relationship between drinking and anxiety, sexual arousal, mood, and motor abilities are also discussed. It is concluded that the ingestion of alcohol produces an indefinite or ambiguous physiological reaction, the interpretation of which appears to be more influenced by prior beliefs, the drinking environment, and personal payoffs than by the physical effects of alcohol.

9. McCarty, D., Diamond, W., & Kaye, M. Alcohol, sexual arousal, and the transfer of excitation. *Journal of Personality and Social Psychology,* 1982, *42,* 977–988.

Investigations of the alcohol-related disinhibition of responses to deviant sexual stimuli suggest that the pharmacological actions of ethanol have little influence on the disinhibition process. The mere belief that alcohol is consumed is sufficient to induce increased sexual arousal. Studies with conventional stimuli, however, suggest that interactions occur between the pharmacological presence of ethanol and the psychological expectations of its presence. Thus, this article examines the contribution of pharmacological, cognitive, and environmental variables to perceived sexual arousal. A balanced-placebo design varied drink instruction and drink content independently. Pictures that elicited either a low or moderate level of self-reported sexual arousal were viewed and evaluated by men (n=64) and women (n=64) after completing their drinks. The evaluations and arousal measures suggested significant Instruction X Content X Arousal interactions. The strongest perceptions of arousal occurred among individuals who did not know they were drinking alcohol (i.e., subjects who were told that their alcoholic drinks did not contain alcohol). Apparently, when drinkers were unaware of the alcohol intoxication, the pharmacological excitation induced by alcohol transferred to the perception and evaluation of the slides. (Author)

10. Millman, R. B., & Khuri, E. T. Adolescence and substance abuse. In J. H. Lowinson & P. Ruiz (Eds.), *Substance abuse: Clinical problems and perspectives.* Baltimore, MD: Williams & Wilkins, 1981.

Adolescents use and/or abuse alcohol more than any other drug. Theories of drug and alcohol abuse assert: (1) that masked depression represented by boredom, restlessness, sexual promiscuity, and other symptoms figures in the etiology of drug abuse; (2) that drugs function in self-treatment of painful emotion; and (3) that youthful drug users are sensation seeking, low in self-esteem and coping skills, more rebellious and impulsive, and less ambitious. Some young people find sexual experiences unsatisfactory due to anxiety or lack of experience. They find that low doses of some drug or alcohol help to relieve inhibitions and to improve performance.

11. Milman, D. H., & Wen-Huey, S. Patterns of drug usage among university students: V. Heavy use of marihuana and alcohol by undergraduates. *College Health*, 1973, *21*, 181–187.

Questionnaire data from 6,110 students was analyzed to examine the correlations between marijuana and alcohol use and factors such as user's gender, age, and marital status; quality of relationship with parents; high school and college performance; and sexual activity. Marijuana and alcohol use was greater among students who were sexually active than among those who were not. Homosexuals were more likely to use both of these drugs than were heterosexuals, with marijuana use being more likely than alcohol use.

12. Renshaw, D. C. Sex and drugs. *South Africa Medical Journal*, 1978, *54*, 322–326.

The following drugs and chemicals are discussed as they relate to sex: alcohol; aphrodisiacs; hormones; stimulants; antidepressants; tranquilizers; hypnotics; antihypertensive drugs, antihistamines, and anticholinergic drugs; marijuana and psychedelic drugs. It is concluded that sexual side effects of needed medications must be not only noted, but carefully and scientifically studied by physicians, since these may offer important avenues of understanding of the many unsolved riddles of the neurophysiology of human sexual response. (NCALI)

13. Rockwell, K., Ellinwood, E., Kantor, C., Maack, W., & Schrumpf, J. Drugs and sex: Scene of ambivalence. *Journal of the American College of Health Association*, 1973, *21*, 483–488.

A survey of the relationship between sex and drug use is reported. Data obtained from questionnaires indicate that 51% of the male and 44% of the female respondents had tried drugs, alcohol, or a combination of both in order to intensify sexual experience.

14. Schuster, R. Zur sexuellen hemmungsfähigkeit bei niedriger blutalkoholkonzentration: Eine experimentelle untersuchung. [Sexual inhibition at low blood alcohol concentrations: An experimental study.] *Beitrage zur Gerichtlichen Medizin*, 1980, *38*, 337–342.

15. Sivochalova, O. V. Otdalennyye posledstviya vozdeistviya alkogolya. [Late sequelae of alcohol exposure.] *Fel'dsher Akusherstvo*, 1979, *44*, 32–34.

Biomedical consequences of alcohol use and abuse, with particular emphasis on the effect of alcohol on sexual functions and genetics, are briefly presented for the purpose of alcohol education of the nursing staff. (RUCAS)

16. Steinglass, P., & Moyer, J. K. Assessing alcohol use in family life: A necessary but neglected area for clinical research. *Family Coordinator*, 1977, *26*, 53–60.

Research into the impact of alcohol use on family life and the relationship between alcohol use and interactional behavior has been minimal. Behavioral science instruments measuring family function, family interaction, or family structure have systematically excluded alcohol use as a significant variable. This paper addresses itself to this oversight in family research methodology. Two representative family studies are reviewed to illustrate how they could have benefited from the inclusion of alcohol-related data. Suggested alterations in methodology are offered to close this "alcohol gap." For example, alcohol-related items could be added to questionnaire instruments in order to ascertain the extent to which each of the various areas of family functioning (e.g., sexual behavior) is alcohol-related. Lastly, the discussion offers several explanations for why alcohol abuse has been so uniformly ignored by family researchers. (Author)

17. Straus, R., & Bacon, S. D. Beliefs about drinking and sexual behavior. In R. Strauss & S. D. Bacon, *Drinking in college*. New Haven, CT: Yale University Press, 1953.

Information about college students' attitudes toward alcohol and drinking as well as their social backgrounds and behavior while drinking was collected from 17,000 students between 1949 and 1951. One chapter is devoted specifically to beliefs about drinking and sexual behavior. Most students associated drinking with some form of sexual activity, expressing such beliefs as that drinking precipitates feelings of sexual excitement and accompanies or facilitates petting. A relationship was found between students' drinking behavior and their endorsement of an association between alcohol and sexual activity such that those who drink more were more likely to make the association. Marital status and religious affiliation, used as indices of sexual experience and moral indoctrination, were also related to beliefs. Actual data on sexual activity were not available. The data are broken down by sex of respondent, and comparisons are made. For instance, female students were slightly less likely than males to associate alcohol with sexual activity and more likely to have no opinion. (RUCAS)

18. Tobias, J. J. The effects of drug use on the sexual activities of suburban youth. *Counseling and Values*, 1973, *17*, 256–259.

Thirteen seminars involving adolescent drinking, drug use, and sexual behavior are presented. Discussion of these leads to the conclusions that drugs, including alochol, appear to: (1) reduce inhibitions, (2) precipitate unpredictable sexual behavior, and (3) offer a socially acceptable excuse for premeditated acts. Scientific exploration of drug use and adolescent behavior is needed.

19. Wilmot, R. Sexual drinking and drift. *Journal of Drug Issues*, 1981, *11*, 1–16.

The author examines interactional changes that occur when alcohol intoxication is sought as part of a sexual scenario. Focus is on a "situation of company," said to occur in relation to sexual drinking, i.e., drinking for a sexual motive, and on how such a situation can equivocate interaction and thereby distort the principles of time, dose, and effect. It is contended that when such a distortion occurs without the full knowledge of the participants, sexual anomie develops. In this light, alcohol can be seen as a sexual talisman rather than a sexual aphrodisiac. (NCALI)

20. Witters, W. L., & Jones-Witters, P. *Drugs and sex*. New York: Macmillan, 1975, 228.

Early use of liquors and cordials was as love potions. Belief in the potion's power plus alcohol's suppression of inhibition produces, for some people, an increase in sexuality. Continued drinking diminishes sexual abilities due to loss of neural control and coordination.

2. Females

21. Lolli, G. Alcohol and the American woman. In G. Lolli, *Social drinking: The effects of alcohol*. New York: Collier Books, 1961.

Women's roles and role confusion lead to problems of sexual adjustment and excessive alcohol use. Confusion about appropriate feminine sexual responses leads to alcohol abuse when alcohol's disinhibiting effects are discovered. Alcohol is then used habitually to achieve the desired sexual responsiveness. The pleasures induced by alcohol become woven into sexual experiences and lead to addictive drinking. Addictive drinking makes a woman more vulnerable to sexual attack and induces a lack of control resulting in less discrimination in choosing a sex partner.

22. Malatesta, V. J., Pollack, R. H., Crotty, T. D., & Peacock, L. J. Acute alcohol intoxication and female orgasmic response. *The Journal of Sex Research*, 1982, *18*, 1–17.

This study tested the hypothesis that increasing levels of acute alcohol intoxication are related to systematic changes in female orgasmic experience reflected by physiological, behavioral, and cognitive indices. Using a repeated measures design with monthly experimental sessions, each of 18 university women was sustained at 4 different blood alcohol concentrations (BAC) in counterbalanced order prior to viewing sexually explicit videotapes and engaging in masturbation to orgasm. Measures of vaginal blood volume obtained by means of a vaginal photoplethysmograph and complemented by a behavioral latency measure showed a progressive and systematic depressant effect of alcohol on orgasmic responding. Higher BACs were associated with longer orgasmic latencies and decreased subjective intensity of orgasm, while paradoxically women reported significantly greater sexual arousal and orgasmic pleasurability under conditions of moderate and high alcohol intoxication. Results have implications for treatment and prevention of alcohol-induced orgasmic dysfunction, and the data suggest that women's orgasms will occur more readily under conditions of no alcohol consumption. Modest intake of alcohol, however, may be expected to result in greater feelings of sexual arousal, a more enjoyable orgasmic experience, and only a moderate increase in the time it takes to reach orgasm. (Author)

23. Saunders, B. Psychological aspects of women and alcohol. In Camberwell Council on Alcoholism, *Women and alcohol*. New York: Tavistock Publications, 1980.

Attempts to consider the psychological factors involved in the use of alcohol by women are confounded by a number of issues, including changing views on alcoholism, which avoid a fixed symptomatology and which make generalization about alcoholics more difficult. It is also likely that, since per capita consumption is rising rapidly and women's drinking is becoming more widely accepted, the woman alcoholic of today and of the future will be different from her historical counterpart of more abstemious decades. Today, however, women are still more moderate and less frequent consumers of alcohol than are men. Drinking by women is often viewed as being associated with promiscuity, or at least with a lessening of sexual restraint. However, this association between drinking and sexual freedom in women has been more alluded to than investigated. Similarities in psychological characteristics of men and women alcoholics may reflect social influences in the development and presentation of alcoholism in women, rather than a greater preexisting psychopathology. The Freudian view of normal, healthy woman as narcissistic, dependent, masochistic, and characterized by inhibited hostility and low self-esteem is no longer considered tenable, and there is scientific evidence that clearly demonstrates that on most variables there are no marked psychological differences between the sexes. Studies of gender identity, locus of control, loss of self-esteem, and sociological factors are not conclusive in demonstrating real differences between men and women. (RUCAS)

24. Sparrow, M. J. Contraception practice of abortion patients. *New Zealand Medical Journal*, 1980, *91*, 104–106.

Of 100 abortion patients in New Zealand, 6 women attributed their nonuse of contraception to alcohol intake and partying. (RUCAS)

25. Wilson, G. T., & Lawson, D. M. Effects of alcohol on sexual arousal in women. *Journal of Abnormal Psychology*, 1976, *85*, 489–497.

In each of 4 weekly experimental sessions 16 female university students (aged 18 to 22), all moderate social drinkers, were given one of 4 doses of alcohol (equivalent to 0.05, 0.25, 0.50, and 0.75 g of alcohol per kg of body weight). Prior to viewing an erotic film depicting an explicit heterosexual interaction and a control film, 8 women were informed on the basis of a bogus questionnaire that alcohol would increase, and 8 were told that it would decrease, their sexual arousal. A self-rating questionnaire answered before viewing the films revealed that only one of the 8 in the decrease-instructional set predicted a decrease, but 5 of the increase-instructional set predicted an increase. With increasing alcohol dose, more women predicted arousal levels in agreement with their instructional set. After the erotic film self-reported sexual arousal increased with alcohol dose, but vaginal pressure pulse measurements, obtained by a vaginal photoplethysmograph, revealed a significant negative linear relationship between increasing doses of alcohol and sexual arousal ($P < .05$). The women in the increase-instructional set exhibited less sexual arousal than those in the decrease-instructional set, results which might be attributed to performance pressure in the experiment. Measurements of muscle tension and the sexual content of the Thematic Apperception Test showed no significant correlations between instructional set, alcohol dose, or vaginal pressure pulse measures. (RUCAS)

26. Wilson, G. T., & Lawson, D. M. Expectancies, alcohol, and sexual arousal in women. *Journal of Abnormal Psychology,* 1978, *87,* 358–367.

A total of 40 university women volunteers, all social drinkers between the ages of 18 and 35 years, were randomly assigned to one of 2 expectancy conditions in which they were led to believe that the beverage they were administered contained either vodka and tonic or tonic only. For half the subjects in each expectancy condition the beverage actually contained vodka; for the other half, tonic only. After their drinks, measures of vaginal pressure pulse obtained by means of a vaginal photoplethysmograph were recorded during a nonerotic control film and 2 erotic films, one depicting heterosexual interaction, the other homosexual interaction. The 2 groups that received alcohol, regardless of whether they believed that their drinks contained alcohol, showed significantly reduced sexual arousal during both erotic films. No effects of expectancy or an interaction between alcohol and expectancy were obtained. The subjects' subjective estimates of intoxication were significantly correlated with their self-report of sexual arousal during both erotic films. We discuss the difference between these results and previous findings using similar procedures with male social drinkers. (Author)

27. Zucker, R. A., Battistich, V. A., & Langer, G. B. Sexual behavior, sex-role adaptation and drinking in young women. *Journal of Studies on Alcohol,* 1981, *42,* 457–465.

A sample of 370 unmarried undergraduate women provided data on: (1) quantity, frequency, and variability of alcohol consumption; (2) ratings of escape motivation for drinking; (3) sexual intercourse and birth control use; (4) relationship permanence; (5) sex-role adaptation using standardized measures, i.e., femininity scale of the California Psychological Inventory, the McClelland and Watts index of sex-typed attitudes and interests, and the Franck Drawing Completion Test; and (6) fantasies in response to a Thematic Apperception Test designed to elicit pregnancy, motherhood, relationship, and sex themes. Heavy-escape drinkers, those who rated 2 or more escape motivations as important and who consumed large amounts of alcohol, were found to be more sexually active and had earlier heterosexual experiences. Few relationships were found between the sex-role measures and alcohol consumption. Data were found to support the hypotheses that: (a) lack of satisfactory affectional interactions among heavy drinkers leads to more sexual activity and (b) self-images and fantasies of heavy drinkers reflect conflict about sex and relationships. The authors conclude that sex-role issues may be epiphenomenally related to women's drinking.

3. Males

28. Barling, J., & Fincham, F. Alcohol, psychological conservatism, and sexual interest in male social drinkers. *Journal of Social Psychology,* 1980, *112,* 135–144.

The present study investigated self-reported sexual interest following alcohol consumption in 48 male social drinkers (mean age = 19.7 years). A sexual interest questionnaire and Wilson's Psychological Conservatism Scale were administered in a pretest-posttest design. The results indicated that while self-reported sexual interest appeared to increase with alcohol doses, beliefs regarding the alcohol content of the drink may mediate this change. Moreover, conservatism and self-reported sexual interest were not significantly related, although the significant negative correlation between the antihedonism factor and sexual interest disappeared when .8 g/kg of alcohol was consumed. (Author)

29. Briddell, D. W. The effects of alcohol and expectancy set on male sexual arousal. (Doctoral dissertation, Rutgers University, The State University of New Jersey, 1975). *Dissertation Abstracts International,* 1975, *36,* 2460B–2461B. (University Microfilms No. 75-24,665)

Forty-eight undergraduate males were assigned to 8 experimental groups. The 6 subjects within each group received one of 4 dose levels of beverage alcohol and one of 2 different sets of expectancy instructions regarding sexual arousal. Changes in penile tumescence, in response to an erotic film, were measured physiologically by a mercury-in-rubber strain gauge. Muscle tension levels were also monitored during the film viewing. In addition, several adjunctive measures of sexual arousal were employed: (a) sexual imagery, (b) the subjective report of arousal, and (c) the estimation of the extent of penile erection. Alcohol significantly reduced the levels of penile tumescence (negative linear relationship). The expectancy instructions regarding alcohol's "effect" did not significantly influence the penile response. Sexual imagery was negatively correlated with penile tumescence, while the subjective reports of sexual arousal and the estimations of penile erection were positively correlated with the physiological measure of sexual arousal. Muscle tension levels were not significantly influenced by alcohol or the expectancy set, nor was muscle tension correlated with penile tumescence. (Author)

30. Briddell, D. W., Rimm, D. C., Caddy, G. R., Krawitz, G., Sholis, D., & Wunderlin, R. J. Effects of alcohol and cognitive set on sexual arousal to deviant stimuli. *Journal of Abnormal Psychology,* 1978, *87,* 418–430.

Forty-eight undergraduate male social drinkers were randomly assigned to one of 2 expectancy set conditions in which they were led to believe that the beverage they were administered contained alcohol or no alcohol. For half of the subjects in each expectancy condition, the beverage was an alcoholic malt liquor; the others drank a nonalcoholic malt beverage. After their drinks, changes in penile tumescence in response to normal and deviant tape recordings and to self-generated fantasy were measured physiologically by a mercury-in-rubber strain gauge. The cognitive set (expectancy) significantly increased penile tumescence in response to the various erotic recordings. Alcohol did not significantly influence levels of sexual arousal. Subjects who believed they had consumed an alcoholic beverage evidenced significantly more arousal to the forcible rape recording and to the sadistic stimuli than subjects who believed that they had consumed a nonalcoholic beverage, regardless of the actual contents of the beverage. The cognitive set, as well as the alcohol, significantly influenced several adjunctive measures of arousal, including heart rate, skin temperature, and subjective reports of sexual arousal. Self-report measures of sexual arousal were positively correlated with penile tumescence. (Author)

31. Briddell, D. W., & Wilson, G. T. Effects of alcohol and expectancy set on male sexual arousal. *Journal of Abnormal Psychology*, 1976, *85*, 225–234.

Forty-eight undergraduate males were assigned to 8 experimental groups. The 6 subjects within each group received one of 4 dose levels of beverage alcohol and one of 2 different sets of expectancy instructions regarding sexual arousal. Changes in penile tumescence, in response to an erotic film, were measured physiologically by a mercury-in-rubber strain gauge. Muscle tension levels were also monitored during the film viewing. In addition, the following adjunctive measures of sexual arousal were employed: (a) sexual imagery, (b) the subjective report of arousal, and (c) the estimation of the extent of penile erection. Alcohol significantly reduced the levels of penile tumescence (negative linear relation). The expectancy instructions regarding alcohol's effect did not significantly influence the penile response. Sexual imagery was negatively correlated with penile tumescence, whereas the subjective reports of sexual arousal and the estimations of penile erection were positively correlated with the physiological measure of sexual arousal. Muscle tension levels were not significantly influenced by alcohol or the expectancy set, nor was muscle tension correlated with penile tumescence. (Author)

32. Carpenter, J. A., & Armenti, N. P. Some effects of ethanol on human sexual and aggressive behavior. In B. Kissin & H. Begleiter (Eds.), *The biology of alcoholism*. New York: Plenum Press, 1971.

This chapter reviews the experimental evidence on the actions of alcohol on sexual and aggressive behavior. Of the studies reviewed, 4 deal with human subjects and each involves examining Thematic Apperception Test (TAT) protocols for the sexual content produced by subjects who had consumed varying amounts of alcohol. In general, alcohol consumption increased sexual imagery on the TAT and resulted in more references to sex in the subjects' conversations while drinking. The authors argue that the findings from both the human and animal studies are not an adequate base for understanding the effects of alcohol on human sexual behavior. One reason is that only male subjects were used in all the studies, animal and human. Also, all studies lacked

criteria for choosing appropriate amounts of alcohol for subjects to consume resulting in some subjects achieving blood alcohol levels that are much higher than would be expected in human social drinking situations. In the studies using dogs, estimated blood alcohol concentration (BAC) ranged from .04% to .44%; using rats, estimated BAC ranged from .29% to .35%; with humans, estimated BAC ranged from .02% to .28%. One difficulty with the human studies was that the meaning of the sexual content on the TAT is unclear both in terms of the process by which the subject arrived at the sexual content (i.e., heightened sensitivity to sexual stimuli) and in the implication for behavior.

33. Clark, R. A. The projective measurement of experimentally induced levels of sexual motivation. *Journal of Experimental Psychology*, 1952, *44*, 391–399.

This study involved the projective measurement of experimentally induced levels of sex motivation. Sexual motivation was aroused by the presentation of slides of nude females in 2 instances and in another instance by the presence of an attractive female. The Thematic Apperception Test (TAT) protocols were analyzed for manifest sex imagery and sex-involved guilt. The results showed that under normal conditions the experimental groups expressed significantly less sex and guilt in the TAT stories than did the control groups. Under conditions of alcohol these results were just the reverse. That is, the experimental group showed significantly more sex and guilt than did the control group. These results are interpreted by assuming that under normal conditions the guilt evoked by sexual arousal is sufficient to inhibit the expression of sex with a consequent lowering of guilt. Under the influence of alcohol, however, the guilt over sexual arousal is reduced enough to permit the expression of sex with a resulting increase in expressed guilt. (Author)

34. Clark, R. A., & Sensibar, M. R. The relationship between symbolic and manifest projections of sexuality with some incidental correlates. *Journal of Abnormal and Social Psychology*, 1955, *50*, 327–334.

Further analyses of data collection in a study reported on previously (*see* entry 33) are presented here. This study involved scoring Thematic Apperception Test (TAT) stories for the presence of sexual symbolism. The stories scored came from 2 different experiments. In one experiment the male subjects were sexually stimulated by viewing photographs of nude women before taking the TAT, while the control group received no such prior stimulation. The second experiment was conducted in the same fashion except that it was carried out in a beer-party atmosphere under the influence of alcohol. The results showed that under nonalcoholic conditions the aroused group expressed significantly more symbolism than the control group. It had been shown previously that this aroused group inhibited the manifest expression of sex. Under conditions of alcohol both groups gave very little symbolism. It had previously been shown that these 2 groups expressed large amounts of manifest sexuality. These results are, of course, in line with the Freudian hypothesis that inhibited sexuality finds an outlet symbolically in fantasy. However, a second, intragroup analysis showing the amount of symbolism, expressed as a function of the amount of manifest sex expressed, revealed the relationship to be curvilinear with both low and high manifest sex corresponding to high symbolism. Various interpretations are discussed for this latter finding. (Author)

35. Conrad, M. E., Perrine, G. M., Barton, J. C., & Durant, J. R. Provoked priapism in sickle cell anemia. *American Journal of Hematology,* 1980, *9,* 121–122.

Two young (aged 19 and 23) Black men with sickle cell anemia developed relative impotence after repeated episodes of priapism. They learned that erection was associated with excessive ingestion of alcohol and utilized this mechanism to satisfy their sexual partners even though this was painful. These episodes were responsible for hospitalization and transfusions required to treat the residual priapism. Several interviews were required in order to learn about the sequence of events leading to this medical problem. This synergistic relationship between alcohol and priapism should be sought in patients with repeated hospitalizations for this complication of sickel cell anemia because it is preventable with appropriate counseling. (RUCAS)

36. Farkas, G. M. *Drugs and sexual response.* Paper presented at the 85th Annual Meeting of the American Psychological Association, San Francisco, August 1977.

This paper presents a brief review of the search for the perfect aphrodisiac, examines some factors to consider when studying drug effects, and comments on the political climate vis-à-vis sex and drug research. A study of the effects of alcohol on male sexual response is also reviewed.

37. Farkas, G. M., & Rosen, R. C. Effect of alcohol on elicited male sexual response. *Journal of Studies on Alcohol,* 1976, *37,* 265–272.

Sexual arousal was measured by changes in penile diameter in 16 young men after consuming alcohol. Subjects had reached up to one of 4 BACs (0.0, 0.025, 0.050, and 0.075) by means of 3 5-minute drinking periods. Penile tumescence was measured by a mercury-in-rubber strain gauge and tonic heart rate was recorded on a Beckman type RM polygraph during the viewing of an erotic film. At the low BAC (0.025) a slight decrease in tumescence rate was found to be associated with the maximum penile diameter increase. At BAC above 0.050 both tumescence rate and diameter were found to diminish rapidly, while tonic heart rate continued to rise as a function of alcohol dose. (RUCAS)

38. Gabel, P. C., Noel, N. E., Keane, T. M., & Lisman, S. A. Effects of sexual versus fear arousal on alcohol consumption in college males. *Behaviour Research and Therapy,* 1980, *18,* 519–526.

To compare the effects of pleasant and aversive arousal on alcohol consumption, 18 male undergraduates had 3 weekly sessions to separately view erotic, mutilation, or neutral slides in a simulated memory experiment. Following exposure to the slides, they received access to alcoholic and nonalcoholic beverages, which were presented to half the subjects in a taste rating task and to half as the result of engaging in an operant lever-press task. Subjects believed these tasks to be distractors during a purported retention interval. Self-report instruments and basal skin conductance confirmed the success of the affective manipulations. However, only the subjects using the taste task after viewing erotic slides significantly increased alcohol consumption. These results question a tension reduction model of drinking and qualify the contribution of autonomic arousal to motivation for drinking. (Author)

39. Johnson, H. J. *Executive life-styles: A Life Extension Institute report on alcohol, sex and health.* New York: Thomas Y. Crowell, 1974.

Approximately 6,000 male executives and businessmen completed a 21-question multiple-choice questionnaire on their habits related to alcohol consumption, sexual behavior, and health. Chapter 11 is devoted specifically to the relationships between sex, alcohol, and health. The author reports that larger numbers of heavy drinkers (those consuming more than 4 ounces of alcohol daily) feel that alcohol enhances their sexual arousal. Alcohol was also associated with incidence of extramarital affairs and divorce.

40. Kalin, R., McClelland, D. C., & Kahn, M. The effects of male social drinking on fantasy. *Journal of Personality and Social Psychology,* 1965, *1,* 441–452.

This article reports on 3 experiments in which a total of 124 college males wrote stories about Thematic Apperception Test (TAT) pictures at 3 points during social drinking, either in living room discussion groups or at stag cocktail parties. Sixty-two comparable subjects wrote under similar conditions when only nonalcoholic beverages were served. In contrast to the control or "dry" subjects whose protocols showed almost no changes, the protocols of the "wet" subjects showed significant increases in various sentient thoughts, particularly with moderate drinking, and decreases in various inhibitory thoughts with heavier drinking. Among the former, meaning contrast and physical aggression thoughts increased up to a maximum at 3–4 drinks (containing 1.5-oz. shots of 86-proof alcoholic beverage). They then decreased and were replaced by an ever increasing number of physical sex thoughts from 6 drinks on. The decreases in inhibitory thoughts—aggression restraint, fear-anxiety, and time concern—occurred regularly only after heavy drinking (from 6 drinks on). Physical aggression thoughts recurred again at high frequency in those subjects who drank very heavily (10 drinks and up). A sentience score based on the preparty TAT, consisting of the sentient categories which increased less some of the inhibitory categories which decreased, predicted the amount of alcohol that would subsequently be consumed. (Author)

41. Lang, A. R., Searles, J., Lauerman, R., & Adesso, V. Expectancy, alcohol, and sex guilt as determinants of interest in and reaction to sexual stimuli. *Journal of Abnormal Psychology,* 1980, *5,* 644–653.

Seventy-two male undergraduate social drinkers were selected from high, moderate, and low scorers on the Sex Guilt subscale of Mosher's Forced-Choice Guilt Inventory.

Equal numbers from each group were randomly assigned to one of 4 conditions in a balanced-placebo design utilized to control for psychological as well as physiological factors determining the effects of drinking on behavior. After consuming their beverages, subjects viewed and evaluated photographic slides of varying erotic content and then reported on their sexual arousal. The time individuals spent viewing each slide was unobtrusively recorded. Overall, greater sexual arousal was indicated by individuals who thought they had received alcoholic beverages, regardless of actual drink content. In all conditions except the high sex guilt/expect tonic groups, viewing times increased as a positive linear function of pornography ratings of the slides. Results are interpreted as demonstrating that psychological aspects of individual differences can mediate expectancy effects in research on alcohol and social behavior. (Author)

42. Lansky, D., & Wilson, G. T. Alcohol, expectations, and sexual arousal in males: An information processing analysis. *Journal of Abnormal Psychology,* 1981, *90,* 35–45.

Using a balanced-placebo drink administration procedure, 48 male social drinkers were presented with erotic and nonerotic stimuli. Selective attention and recognition memory were measured in both visual and auditory modalities; penile tumescence was recorded continuously in response to auditory stimuli. The belief that alcohol had been consumed increased penile tumescence to both heterosexual and homosexual stimuli, but only in subjects high in sex guilt. Mild intoxication itself had no effect. Alcohol impaired memory for visual stimuli, while the belief that alcohol had been drunk facilitated memory for stimuli in the auditory modality. Correlational analysis did not support the hypothesis that alcohol expectation's impact on sexual responsiveness is mediated directly through its influence on selective attention and memory processes. (Author)

43. Malatesta, V. J. The effects of alcohol on ejaculation latency in human males. (Doctoral dissertation, University of Georgia, 1978). *Dissertation Abstracts International,* 1978, *40,* 3558B. (University Microfilms No. 79-01,664)

This research represents an initial attempt to investigate systematically the effects of various levels of alcohol intoxication on the orgasmic-ejaculatory response in human males. Twenty-four adult male volunteers, between the ages of 22 and 34, were sustained at one of 4 blood alcohol concentrations (0.0, 0.03, 0.06, 0.09% ± .005%) during 4 separate counterbalanced experimental sessions, preceded by a desensitization session. With the subsequent onset of sexually explicit stimuli, subjects were asked to masturbate to ejaculation. The dependent measures thus consisted of: ejaculation latency as measured by an electromyographic recording technique and supplemented by a voluntary temporal response measure; heart-rate measures at levels of resting, orgasmic, and difference thresholds; and subjective responses to a postexperimental questionnaire. The results indicated that increasing levels of alcohol intoxication showed significant degradation in male masturbatory effectiveness. Increasing

levels of alcohol intoxication were associated with: significant increases in ejaculation latency, significant decreases in reported sexual arousal, a significant incidence of reported difficulty in attaining orgasm, and significantly decreased pleasurability and intensity of orgasm. (Author)

44. Malatesta, V. J., Pollack, R. H., Wilbanks, W. A., & Adams, H. E. Alcohol effects on the orgasmic-ejaculatory response in human males. *The Journal of Sex Research,* 1979, *15,* 101–107.

Increasing levels of alcohol intoxication, as measured by blood alcohol concentration, produced significant degradation in male masturbatory effectiveness. Employing psychophysiological indices of orgasm and several subjective criteria, a progressive and systematic effect of alcohol on the orgasmic-ejaculatory response was found. Results are discussed with implications for the etiology, treatment, and prevention of alcohol-induced sexual dysfunction in males. (Author)

45. Masters, W. H., & Johnson, V. E. *Human sexual response.* Boston: Little Brown, 1966, 267–269.

Many males experience their first erectile failure while under the influence of alcohol. Secondary impotence may result due to excessive performance concerns. Among men in their late 40s or early 50s, secondary impotence is more highly associated with excessive alcohol consumption than any other single factor.

46. McClelland, D. C., Davis, W. N., Kalin, R., & Wanner, E. *The drinking man.* New York: The Free Press, 1972.

This book reports on 10 years of the authors' research into the role of alcohol in human life, guided by the premise that alcohol consumption is a psychologically motivated act. Concerns with sexuality and interest in participating in sexual behavior are among the motivational variables examined. Subjects are mostly male college students. Methodology makes extensive use of Thematic Apperception Test productions. The authors conclude that the need for power is the primary motivator of excessive drinking. Sexual themes in response to projective tests are classified as indicants of need for power.

47. Montague, D. K., James, R. E., Jr., De Wolfe, V. G., & Martin, L. M. Diagnostic evaluation, classification, and treatment of men with sexual dysfunction. *Urology,* 1979, *14,* 545–548.

In a detailed evaluation of sexual dysfunction in 165 men who were also asked about their alcohol intake, only one was found whose dysfunction was primarily due to excessive alcohol intake. (RUCAS)

48. Rubin, H. B., & Henson, D. E. Effects of alcohol on male sexual responding. *Psychopharmacology,* 1976, *47,* 123–134.

Alcohol had a dose-related depressive effect on male sexual arousal elicited by erotic motion pictures, but only the highest of 3 test doses had a depressive effect on the ability to become aroused in the absence of overt stimuli. Low (0.5 or 0.6 ml/kg) or moderate (1.0 or 1.2 ml/kg) doses of alcohol caused a small but significant depression of mean sexual arousal, but other measures of sexual response were not affected. Large (1.5 or 1.8 ml/kg) doses significantly depressed both evoked arousal and arousal in the absence of overt erotic stimuli. By contrast, none of the 3 doses significantly impaired the subjects' ability to voluntarily inhibit their arousal by the films, even though some deterioration in this ability was experienced after the moderate dosage. The effects of alcohol on sexual response were not correlated with its effects on a nonsexual matching task, to subjective reports on the effect of alcohol on sexual behavior, or to reported drinking history.

49. Tamerin, J. S., & Mendelson, J. H. The psychodynamics of chronic inebriation: Observations of alcoholics during the process of drinking in an experimental group setting. *American Journal of Psychiatry,* 1969, *125,* 58–71.

Four male volunteer alcoholic subjects were studied prior to, during, and following a period of experimentally induced intoxication. The subjects were restricted to a closed research unit for 10 weeks. The study consisted of: a 2-week observation period, a 3-week period of programmed alcohol administration, a 10-day withdrawal period, a 3-week period of free-access drinking, and a final 10-day withdrawal period prior to discharge. During states of intoxication there was a marked increase in sexual feelings and activities in direct and derivative forms. With the onset of intoxication, a striking upsurge of loving feelings emerged. There was also an increase in heterosexual interest. The predominant sexual activity, however, was homosexual, expressed in disguised form as playfulness and helpfulness.

50. Tamerin, J. S., Weiner, S., & Mendelson, J. H. Alcoholics' expectancies and recall of experiences during intoxication. *The American Journal of Psychiatry,* 1970, *126,* 39–46.

Using a modified Q-sort test administered to 13 male alcoholics, the authors attempted to assess alcoholics' expectancies prior to drinking and to compare these with their subsequent self-reports of feeling states and behavior during experimentally induced intoxication. They found that during intoxication subjects observed significantly more aggression, sexuality, and dysphoria in themselves than they had anticipated. A marked increase in irresponsible behavior, however, was successfully predicted. (Author)

51. Van Thiel, D. H. Sexual effect of alcohol. *Medical Aspects of Human Sexuality,* 1979, *13,* 66.

In the question and answer section of the journal, the author responds to a question on the paradoxical effect of alcohol on sexuality (i.e., enhanced sexual arousal with ingestion of alcohol accompanied by interference with performance with increasing amounts of alcohol) and states that the central nervous system depressant effect of alcohol progresses sequentially beginning with higher cortical functioning which is responsibile for superego control of sexual behavior. The CNS depressant effect then proceeds to the level of the cortex responsible for sexual arousal and potency as more alcohol is ingested.

52. Westling, A. On the correlation of the consumption of alcoholic drinks with some sexual phenomenon of Finnish male students. *International Journal of Sexology,* 1954, *7,* 109–115.

A questionnaire answered by 893 male Finnish students showed that the beginning of sexual activity in the form of ejaculation or masturbation did not correlate with subsequent consumption of alcohol. Alcohol consumption and age at which first intoxication occurred, however, were correlated to initial extramarital sexual intercourse. Students whose first intoxication occurred between 13 and 15 started their premarital intercourse at the average age of 17.8, while those whose first intoxication occurred at 22 had their first extramarital intercourse at 25. The younger the age at which the first alcohol intoxication occurs or the greater the consumption of alcohol, the higher is the cumulative incidence of premarital intercourse. These results cannot be generalized, for various factors, such as customs of population groups, are influential. Nevertheless the study again shows the old connection between wine and love: "Sine Cerere et Baccho friget Venus" (Terence) or "Wo Bacchus einzieht da sitzt Frau Venus hinter dem Ofen" (Tobben). (RUCAS)

53. Wilson, G. T., & Lawson, D. M. Expectancies, alcohol, and sexual arousal in male social drinkers. *Journal of Abnormal Psychology,* 1976, *85,* 587–594.

The effects of expectation of alcohol intake on sexual arousal were studied in 40 undergraduate men, all social drinkers (aged 18 to 22), by informing them that they were receiving either vodka (in doses of 0.5 g of alcohol per kg of body weight) and tonic or tonic only, while actually giving the expected beverage to only half of each group; the rest were given the other beverage. Penile tumescence was measured by a penile strain gauge during 2 erotic films of an explicit heterosexual or male homosexual interaction. While no significant effects of alcohol were found, those who believed they had consumed alcohol had greater increases in penile tumescence during both films than those who believed they had taken tonic only. No significant correlations were found between penile tumescence and forehead temperature during the films or sexual content of the Thematic Apperception Test or of the Word Association Test administered before the films; postfilm self-reports of sexual arousal were positively correlated with penile tumescence. (RUCAS)

54. Wilson, G. T., Lawson, D. M., & Abrams, D. B. Effects of alcohol on sexual arousal in male alcoholics. *Journal of Abnormal Psychology,* 1978, *87,* 609–616.

During successive daily sessions, each of 8 chronic male alcoholics received, in counterbalanced order, 4 doses of beverage alcohol prior to viewing nonerotic and erotic films. Measures of penile tumescence obtained by means of a penile plethysmograph showed a significant negative linear effect of increasing alcohol doses during the heterosexual and homosexual films. Subjects' expectations about the effect of alcohol on sexual arousal and behavior were discrepant with these physiological findings. Consistently, subjects reported that alcohol would have no effect on their sexual arousal or would increase it. (Author)

4. Alcohol as an Aphrodisiac

55. Benedek, T. G. Food and drink as aphrodisiacs. *Sexual Behavior,* 1972, *2,* 5–10.

The use of plant and animal products for aphrodisiac effects is discussed in historical perspective. In earliest history, alcoholic beverages served as a vehicle for administering aphrodisiac preparations. For instance, in Babylon the cure for impotence was prepared in beer. Use of alcohol in this fashion increased during the 9th century A.D. with the discovery of distillation. Aphrodisiac properties were attributed to alcohol in its own right which was recorded as early as the 12th century A.D. As knowledge about nutrition and situational influences on sexuality and sexual performance has accumulated, aphrodisiac effects are attributed more to the eating and drinking of healthful food in a relaxed setting than to the specific foods or drinks (e.g., alcohol) consumed.

56. Burgoyne, D. Sexual effect of small quantities of alcohol. *Medical Aspects of Human Sexuality,* 1976, *10,* 9.

The author responds to a reader's question about the effectiveness of alcohol as an aphrodisiac in the question and answer section of this journal. He indicates that alcohol is basically a central nervous system depressant and, therefore, not actually an aphrodisiac. The apparent aphrodisiac effect depends upon the quantity of alcohol consumed and the emotional condition of the patient at the time. The disinhibiting effect of small amounts of alcohol may be sufficiently calming to the individual to allow him/her to be stimulated more easily and to function more effectively in a sexual encounter. With continued consumption of alcohol, the sedative effect will be felt; and the individual will find it more and more difficult to be stimulated and to respond effectively. The effects of alcohol can dull the senses and work in the opposite direction from an aphrodisiac.

57. Bush, P. J. *Drugs, alcohol, and sex.* New York: Richard Marek Publishers, 1980.

This book for the educated layperson addresses the aphrodisiac and anaphrodisiac effects of recreational drugs and prescribed and over-the-counter medicines. The information on alcohol was gathered from medical, psychological, and other research journals, as well as from a questionnaire completed by approximately 250 volunteers recruited by newspaper ads, word of mouth, and distribution at an annual meeting of the American Pharmaceutical Association. Members of a community of former drug addicts also volunteered. The questionnaire evaluated drug use and changes in sexual function associated with the drug use. Although alcohol is discussed in a variety of places throughout the book, one chapter, devoted entirely to alcohol, discusses the disinhibiting effect of small amounts of alcohol, which can facilitate

sexual functioning, contrasting this with the disruptive effects of increasing doses and the dysfunction caused by chronic alcoholism. These observations are illustrated with comments made by male and female questionnaire respondents and supported by reviews of literature on laboratory studies. In addition, the chapter touches on homosexuality and alcoholism, sexual crimes, and the role of expectations for sexual arousal under the influence of alcohol. Use of alcohol in conjunction with various other drugs, historical comments, and long-term effects on sexual physiology are contained in other chapters of the book.

58. Edwards, R. The use of drugs in the search for a human aphrodisiac experience. *Journal of Drug Education,* 1971, *1,* 137–145.

This article delineates the search for sexual pleasure through the aid of drugs and other substances. While myths prevail that drugs create the sexually libertine spirit, scientific evidence indicates that no known drug serves as an aphrodisiac. Alcohol and other drugs may be used in moderate doses to free sexual desire temporarily, lower inhibitions, and reduce anxiety. A drug, however, cannot by itself cause individuals to engage in sexual behavior that would otherwise be abhorrent to them. Excessive use of drugs usually is accompanied by diminished sexual interest and performance. L-Dopa and P.C.P.A. are the latest substances used where there have been claims of improvement in human sexual response. The reputed causal relationship between drugs and sex, however, appears to be inconsistent and quite secondary to psychological and emotional factors. (Author)

59. Gallant, D. M. The effect of alcohol and drug abuse on sexual behavior. *Medical Aspects of Human Sexuality,* 1968, *2,* 30–36.

Historically, it appears that people have never been satisfied with their sexual potency. The search for an aphrodisiac can be traced back to the ancient Egyptians. Aphrodisiacs have no objective properties that truly prolong or enhance the sexual act. They do, however, possess properties of olfactory stimulation, gustatory stimulation, and muscular relaxation that may provide secondary enhancement of sexual excitement. Drugs have no true aphrodisiac qualities although they may contribute to grandiose feelings of marked sexual prowess. Alcohol has had a strong association with sexual behavior for thousands of years. Drunkenness offers an opportunity to release inner feelings without fear. The supposed aphrodisiac effect of alcohol may be attributed to the reduction of anxiety about sexual behavior accompanied by muscle relaxation. Excessive consumption has a tendency to repress sexual drives, sometimes to the degree of anesthesia. Acute secondary impotence is frequently caused by and can become a chronic problem as a result of subsequent feelings of inadequacy. Sex therapy must make sobriety a prerequisite to acceptance for treatment.

60. Gay, G. R., Newmeyer, J. A., Elion, R. A., & Wieder, S. Drug-sex practice in the Haight-Ashbury or ''the sensuous hippie.'' In M. Sandler & G. L. Gessa

(Eds.), *Sexual behavior: Pharmacology and biochemistry*. New York: Raven Press, 1975.

Questionnaire data were collected from 59 men and 36 women who were clients of the Haight-Ashbury Free Medical Clinic. Marijuana was the drug most frequently used intentionally to enhance sex. Alcohol, tobacco, cocaine, and heroin played a lesser role but figured significantly in the subjects' sexual-enhancement routine. Some drugs were noted to decrease sexual activity; prominently mentioned were barbiturates, methoqualone, heroin, and large doses of amphetamine or alcohol. The effect of alcohol is definitely dose related.

61. Gay, G. R., & Sheppard, C. W. Sex in the "drug culture." *Medical Aspects of Human Sexuality,* 1972, *6,* 28–47.

A report of the sexual activities of drug abusers, conducted among patients at the Haight-Ashbury Free Medical Clinic, is presented. Results indicate that the sex act itself was seldom reported to be enhanced by alcohol; rather, the effect most often reported was one of disinhibition. While disinhibition was seen at low alcohol levels, with increasing dosage the predominant effect was described as loss of potency. The effects of marijuana, barbiturates, cocaine, LSD, mescaline, psilocybin, and heroin on sexual activity are also included. The dangers of confusing cause-and-effect relationships between drugs and sexual behavior are reviewed. (NCALI)

62. Gay, G. R., & Sheppard, C. W. "Sex-crazed dope fiends"—myth or reality? *Drug Forum,* 1973, *2,* 125–140.

Fifty patients at the Haight-Ashbury Free Clinic, ranging in age from 18 to 30 years, were interviewed regarding their sex-drug practices. Drug use was defined as "more than merely experimental" (i.e., extended daily use of barbiturates or alcohol, multiple occasions of marijuana use, psychedelic trips, and intravenous amphetamine use). Only 4 of the 50 felt that alcohol enhanced their sexual experiences. Alcohol, usually wine, was often taken with marijuana, and the disinhibitory effects of both drugs were repeatedly mentioned in breaking down sexual barriers. In high doses, alcohol was reported to decrease desire and interfere with performance.

63. Griffith, E. F. Alcohol and sex. *The British Journal of Inebriety,* 1938, *36,* 57–60.

That alcohol is a sexual stimulant must be recognized by everyone. That its effect as such is beneficial is a far more debatable point. Alcohol acts mainly on the cerebral centers, thereby arousing sex desire and diminishing sex inhibitions. The judicious use of alcohol in the view of some is considered advantageous under certain circumstances, such as in those cases where there is an excessive nervousness or dread of coitus, or where it is difficult for the woman to obtain orgasm. Where alcohol is needed as an aphrodisiac there is

usually an underlying emotional disturbance or lack of technique. Two case histories are given as illustrations. (Author)

64. Jarvik, M. E., & Brecker, E. M. Drugs and sex: Inhibition and enhancement effects. In J. Money & H. Musaph (Eds.), *Handbook of Sexology.* New York: *Excerpta Medica,* 1977.

In the search for drugs to stimulate or suppress sexuality, both inert and pharmacologically active substances have been imbued with the power to control sexuality. The authors compare folklore about aphrodisiacs with the knowledge gained from contemporary scientific inquiry. Alcohol is among the substances discussed in this context.

65. La-Marca, D. Alcohol and sexuality: The myths and facts surrounding alcohol. In E. J. Tongue (Ed.), *Papers presented at the 24th International Institute on the Prevention and Treatment of Alcoholism.* Lausanne: International Council on Alcohol and Addictions, 1978.

This paper reviews literature pertaining to the myth of the aphrodisiac effects of alcohol. Conclusions from studies indicating the disinhibiting effects of small amounts of alcohol and the dysfunctional effects of large amounts of alcohol were discussed. The paper notes that among males increased and prolonged alcohol abuse leads to impotence that may become permanent. Among females, excessive alcohol consumption is associated with anorgasmia and avoidance of sexual contact. The author points out the need for adequately informed professionals in the field of alcoholism treatment and the need for adequate treatment of alcohol-related sexual dysfunction.

66. MacDougald, D., Jr. Aphrodisiacs and anaphrodisiacs. In A. Ellis & A. Abarbanel (Eds.), *Encyclopedia of Sexual Behavior.* New York: Hawthorn Books, 1967.

The author provides a historical perspective on aphrodisiacs and discusses possible reasons for attributing aphrodisiac properties to some foods, drink, and drugs. Alcohol, by dilating the blood vessels, imparts a sensation of warmth to parts of the body, including the genitals. The narcotic effects of alcohol on the brain tend to remove moral blocks and bring on a light-hearted, often reckless and sexually responsive, state of mind.

67. Selden, G. *Aphrodisia: A guide to sexual food, herbs, and drugs.* New York: E. P. Dutton, 1979.

The book focuses on internal aphrodisiacs, i.e., foods and drugs. Specifically, alcohol is described as "the most common social lubricant in nearly every known culture . . . by far the worst, but still the most popular, the universally proverbial prelude to seduction." Its use throughout written history is reviewed. Sex differences in the effects of alcohol on sexual behavior are described, including a discussion of the relation between inebriation and sexual violence.

B. Effects of Alcohol on Sex Hormones

1. Individuals without Cirrhosis

a. Females

68. Jones, B. M., & Jones, M. K. Women and alcohol: Intoxication, metabolism, and the menstrual cycle. In M. Greenblatt & M. A. Schuckit (Eds.), *Alcoholism problems in women and children.* New York: Grune & Stratton, 1976.

In this review chapter, the authors discuss their research and make comparisons to similar research done by others. In general, it has been found that women's blood alcohol levels (BAL) are higher than men's with equal doses of ethanol per body weight. Blood alcohol levels may vary over the menstrual cycle as a function of steroid levels. Findings are not consistent across studies, and there is a need for more similar research. The authors point out the implications for sexual behavior, reporting an observation made by the experimenters while testing the participants. The subjects commented on an unexpected occurrence, a sensation of sexual excitation at approximately .04% BAL on the ascending limb. The sensation was usually reported as a feeling of clitoral tingling or itching with a warm sensation spreading through the groin area. The sensation dissipated in 10–15 minutes. It was often intense and did not occur in each drinking session.

69. McNamee, B., Grant, J., Ratcliffe, J., Ratcliffe, W., & Oliver, J. Lack of effect of alcohol on pituitary-gonadal hormones in women. *British Journal of Addictions,* 1979, *74,* 316–317.

Ingestion of alcohol (2.8 ml per kg of body weight as vodka) that produced blood alcohol levels of 25.6 ± 1.5 mmol/1 (117.8 ± 7.0 mg/100 ml) 1 to 2 hours after administration caused no changes in: serum testosterone, prolactin or luteinizing hormone, progesterone, estradiol, or follicle-stimulating hormone in 8 healthy women (aged 20–38; mean age 28) in the early follicular phase of the menstrual cycle. The women had no history of alcohol abuse or use of oral contraceptives. Findings point to the possible danger of generalizing about the biological effects of alcohol from research carried out almost entirely on men. (RUCAS)

b. Males

70. Alcohol affects sexuality. *Research Resources Reporter,* January/February 1980.

In a discussion of alcohol's effects on sexuality it is concluded that alcoholic men are slowly and irreversibly de-masculinizing themselves by continuing to drink excessive amounts of alcohol. A biochemical mechanism which causes alcoholic males to exhibit secondary sex characteristics is described. The ease with which infertility caused by alcohol abuse can be diagnosed is stressed. (NCALI)

71. Anylian, G. H., Dorn, J., & Swerdlow, J. The manifestations, aetiology and assessment of ethanol-induced hangover. *South African Medical Journal,* 1978, *54,* 193–198.

This review article focuses on the hangover following ingestion of alcoholic beverages. In general, alcoholic drinks rich in congeners (e.g., whiskey) induce more severe hangover than drinks which are nearly pure diluted alcohol (e.g., vodka). It is probable that alcohol alone in large doses is capable of inducing severe hangover. Treatment of hangover symptoms has been of questionable effectiveness. Detailed studies must be preceded by the development of a system for measurement of hangover symptoms. Scales used in studies of drug treatment of hangover are described. Attention is drawn to the changes in hormone levels, notably aldosterone, renin, cortisol, and testosterone, in males during hangover. The relationship of observed changes in hormone level to hangover symptoms remains obscure.

72. Doorenbos, H. Endocrinologische aspecten van alcoholgebruik. [Endocrinological aspects of alcohol consumption.] *Nederlands Tijdschrift Voor Geneeskunde,* 1979, *123,* 1269–1272.

Alcohol's effects on fat and carbohydrate metabolism and adrenal, gonadal, and other endocrine functions are briefly discussed. (RUCAS)

73. Fabre, L. F., Jr., Pasco, P. J., Liegel, J. M., & Farmer, R. W. Abnormal testosterone excretion in men alcoholics. *Quarterly Journal of Studies on Alcohol,* 1973, *34,* 57–63.

Urinary testosterone glucuronide and 17-ketosteroids were measured in 20 male alcoholics, aged 25 to 45, with no physical signs of gynecomastia or testicular atrophy and with normal liver function, who had been abstinent for 2 weeks and were receiving no medication, and in nonalcoholics of approximately the same age. After several urine samples had been collected at 24-hour intervals, 10 alcoholics were allowed ad libitum consumption of alcoholic beverages for 6 days during continued urine collection. The nondrinking alcoholics' testosterone glucuronide excretion averaged

153.08 μg per 24 hours, significantly different from the 36.7 μg per 24 hours of 11 nonalcoholics (p<.001). The excretion rates of the nondrinking and drinking alcoholics were not significantly different although they tended to be higher after drinking. Androsterone excretion was 0.43 mg per 24 hours in the drinking alcoholics, at a mean blood alcohol concentration of 148 mg per 100 ml (range, 27.5–240), 0.95 in the abstaining alcoholics, and 1.42 in 8 controls. Etiocholanolone excretion was 0.29, 0.71, and 0.63, respectively. Dehydroepiandrosterone excretion was less than 0.01 mg per 24 hours in the 2 groups of alcoholics and 0.47 in the controls. The increased excretion of testosterone glucuronide in alcoholics suggests that there is an increased hepatic conversion of 17-ketosteroids to testosterone and its conjugated metabolites, and that androgen metabolism is shifted from oxidative to reductive pathways.

74. Gordon, G. G., Altman, K., Southren, A. L., Rubin, E., & Lieber, C. S. Effect of alcohol (ethanol) administration on sex-hormone metabolism in normal men. *New England Journal of Medicine,* 1976, *295,* 793–797.

To determine whether ethanol per se affects testosterone metabolism, alcohol was administered to normal male volunteers for periods up to 4 weeks, resulting in an initial dampening of the episodic bursts of testosterone secretion followed by decreases in both the mean plasma concentration and the production rate of testosterone. The volunteers received adequate nutrition and none lost weight during the study, which tended to exclude a nutritional disturbance as the cause of the decreased testosterone levels. The changes in plasma luteinizing hormone suggested both a central (hypothalamus-pituitary) and gonadal effect of alcohol. In addition, alcohol consumption increased the metabolic clearance rate of testosterone in most subjects studied, probably owing to the combined effects of a decreased plasma binding capacity for the androgen and increased hepatic testosterone A-ring reductase activity. These results indicate that alcohol markedly affects testosterone metabolism independently of cirrhosis or nutritional factors. (Author)

75. Gordon, G. G., Southren, A. L., & Lieber, C. S. The effects of alcoholic liver disease and alcohol ingestion on sex hormone levels. *Alcoholism: Clinical and Experimental Research,* 1978, *2,* 259–263.

This article reviews some previously reported data and presents data from a study of 9 healthy young men hospitalized for purposes of the study. Subjects were given controlled doses of alcohol for up to 26 days. Blood was collected at ½-hour to 1-hour intervals for 24-hour periods to be analyzed for testosterone and luteinizing hormone (LH). This study showed that alcohol significantly decreases plasma testosterone levels, with changes noted as early as the first day of alcohol use (loss of pulsatile secretion). This effect is due, in part, to a direct testicular action since it occurred without LH suppression and in the presence of elevated LH levels. More chronic use of alcohol resulted in a suppression of LH. Thus, alcohol use in nonalcoholic men is associated with an effect both at the testicular and hypothalamic-pituitary levels.

76. Gordon, G. G., Southren, A. L., & Lieber, C. S. Hypogonadism and feminization in the male: A triple effect of alcohol. *Alcoholism: Clinical and Experimental Research,* 1979, *3,* 210–212.

This editorial reviews evidence arguing that alcohol has a triple effect on the male endocrine system: (1) reduction of plasma testosterone levels through action at the hypothalamic-pituitary level, (2) alteration of gonadal functioning resulting in lower plasma testosterone, and (3) alcohol mediated alterations of enzyme activities in organs concerned with steroid metabolism. These hypotheses were developed to explain decreased plasma testosterone observed following alcohol ingestion in the absence of alcoholic liver disease. The actions of alcohol at the hypothalamic-pituitary and gonadal level, the dual effect, are supported by considerable evidence. The dual effect, however, does not explain all the observed hormonal changes, e.g., plasma testosterone levels may not drop with acute alcohol ingestion, as the dual effect alone would predict. The expected effect may be mitigated by the increased availability of dihydrotestosterone, a metabolite of testosterone used by the prostate. The availability of dihydrotestosterone is increased by the accelerated conversion by hepatic 5α-reductases of testosterone associated with alcohol consumption. Prolonged alcohol ingestion is associated with a decrease in this enzyme activity, thus accentuating the effects of lowered plasma testosterone and contributing to alcohol-related hypogonadism.

77. Huttunen, M. O., Härkönen, M., Niskanen, P., Leino, T., & Ylikahri, R. Plasma testosterone concentrations in alcoholics. *Journal of Studies on Alcohol,* 1976, *37,* 1165–1177.

Plasma concentrations of testosterone (T) and luteinizing hormone (LH) were studied: (1) during a 4-day withdrawal period in 17 men (mean age 40.5) hospitalized after drinking bouts of 2 to 8 weeks; (2) in 16 skid row alcoholics (men, mean age 50.1) who were actively drinking; and (3) in 16 men controls (social drinkers) matched by age with the skid row alcoholics. Upon admission to the hospital, the alcoholic patients were all given equivalent doses of alcohol to bring them to the same phase of withdrawal for test purposes. Blood samples were taken at 0, 4, 8, 12, 16, 20, 38, and 86 hours after the alcohol dose. A single blood sample was taken from the skid row men and controls. All samples were tested for plasma T and LH; the 17 patients were also tested for blood alcohol concentrations and for the intensity of withdrawal symptoms when each blood sample was taken. Among the patients, levels of plasma T and LH were always within normal range. Testosterone concentrations, however, were significantly lower during the first 2 days of the withdrawal period than toward the end (p<.01). The level of LH was highest at 4 hours after the alcohol dose, with a gradual decrease toward the end of the withdrawal period. There was no correlation between the severity of the withdrawal symptoms and LH levels. Plasma T concentrations among the 16 skid row alcoholics were in the same range as in the controls. Mean LH concentrations were higher (p<.01) among the skid rowers than among the controls. Because plasma T levels were found to be normal among both the skid row men and the alcoholic patients, this study does not support other findings suggesting that gynecomastia and testicular atrophy among some alcoholics would be caused by the direct effects of alcohol on steroid metabolism.

78. Lester, R., Eagon, P. K., & Van Thiel, D. H. Feminization of the alcoholic: The estrogen/testosterone ratio (E/T). *Gastroenterology*, 1979, *76*, 415–417.

The significance of the estrogen/testosterone ratio as it applies to chronic alcoholic men who show hypogonadism and hyperestrogenization is discussed. Alcoholism results in destruction of the male gonad, with diminished plasma testosterone levels. The low plasma testosterone stimulates the activity of estrogen-binding proteins, which could result in increased sensitivity to plasma estrogen. The hypothesis that an individual with a low testosterone and normal or only moderately evaluated estrogen level might become hyperestrongenized is examined. The authors conclude that the current therapy of administering testosterone enanthate to the hypoandrogenized alcoholic male should be considered experimental until it is shown whether or not testosterone administration will decrease hyperestrogenization. (NCALI)

79. Liegel, J. M., Fabre, L. F., Jr., Howard, P. Y., & Farmer, R. W. Plasma testosterone and sex hormone binding globulin (SBG) in alcoholic subjects. *The Physiologist*, 1972, *15*, 198.

Previously, the laboratory reported increased urinary testosterone glucuronide excretion and decreased individual 17-ketosteroid excretion in alcoholic male subjects with normal liver function. This report concerns plasma testosterone and SBG measurements in this population. Plasma testosterone was within normal limits (557 ± 49.6 ng%, $\overline{X}\pm SE$) in abstaining alcoholics ($508+43.8$ ng%), decreased during drinking [blood ETOH (ethanol) 100–200 mg% (387 ± 68.0 ng%)], and increased during withdrawal (802 ± 111.5 ng%) compared with age-paired controls. SBG was significantly ($p<.01$) elevated in male alcoholics ($1/p = .404\pm.071$) as compared to normal males ($1/p = .219\pm.028$), but not ($p<.01$) to normal female values ($1/p = .624\pm.071$). During ETOH consumption no changes were noted. *In vitro*, ETOH (100–200 mg%) decreased protein binding in normal male and female sera. This factor may be related to the decrease in plasma testosterone during drinking. The phenomena observed here may be related to the decreased "maleness" clinically observed in male alcoholics. (Author)

80. Lindholm, J., Fabricius-Bjerre, N., Bahnsen, M., Boiesen, P., Hagen, C., & Christensen, T. Sex steroids and sex-hormone binding globulin in males with chronic alcoholism. *European Journal of Clinical Investigation*, 1978, *8*, 273–276.

Thirty men with chronic alcoholism were studied. Biopsies of the liver and testis were performed in all. Serum concentrations were determined for (a) total and nonprotein bound (free) testosterone and estradiol, (b) dihydrotestosterone and (c) sex-hormone-binding globulin (SHBG). Testosterone and dihydrotestosterone concentrations were normal in most

patients, whereas estradiol and free estradiol were above normal in approximately 50% of the patients. None of the hormones measured differed significantly between patients with and without cirrhosis. SHBG was significantly higher in men with severely reduced spermatogenesis compared to those with intact germinal epithelium, but there was no difference between men with and without cirrhosis. No relation could be demonstrated between clinical signs of hypogonadism and any of the hormones measured. The results support the view that hormonal and sexual disturbances may occur in chronic alcoholism independent of the presence of liver disease. (Author)

81. Linnoila, M., Prinz, P. N., Wonsowicz, C. J., & Leppaluoto, J. Effect of moderate doses of ethanol and phenobarbital on pituitary and thyroid hormones and testosterone. *British Journal of Addiction*, 1980, *75*, 207–212.

Effects of ingestion of .8 g/kg of body weight of ethanol or 100 mg of phenobarbital for 7 consecutive nights on plasma luteinizing hormone (LH), thyroid-stimulating hormone (TSH), prolactin, thyroid hormone (T_3, T_4), and testosterone levels were studied in 5 healthy young men. Ethanol increased plasma TSH levels during sleep whereas phenobarbital decreased plasma TSH levels during sleep and awake periods. Neither ethanol nor phenobarbital had significant effects on plasma prolactin, total T_3, T_4, or testosterone levels. (Author)

82. Lox, C. D., Peddicord, O., Heine, M. W., & Messiha, F. S. The influence of chronic long term alcohol abuse on testosterone secretion in men and rats. *Procedures of the Western Pharmacological Society*, 1978, *21*, 299–302.

In this study, chronic long-term human and rat alcoholics were evaluated for endocrine function as a correlate of ethanol ingestion. Blood samples of 14 chronic alcoholic human males were analyzed for serum testosterone, serum luteinizing hormone (LH), prolactin, and blood alcohol. Blood samples were drawn for court-ordered evaluation of extent of intoxication during admission to a detoxification program. Patients were in various stages of withdrawal or intoxication, including stuperous, and all had long histories of alcohol abuse. Decreased testosterone levels were observed in 50% of the alcoholic men. No significant correlation was found between blood ethanol and testosterone. A significant decrease in circulating LH was found in those individuals with low testosterone. This finding plus the significant relationship between blood alcohol and LH suggest site of action at the hypothalamic-pituitary level.

83. Majumdar, S. K. The effect of chlormethiazole on serum gonadotrophins and testosterone in chronic alcoholics. *Current Medical Research and Opinion*, 1979, *6*, 213–216.

Individual mean serum luteinizing hormone and follicle-stimulating hormone levels in 7 male alcoholics (aged 31–69) were normal, but serum testosterone concentrations were slightly higher than normal, on admission and following treatment with chlormethiazole for 6 days. During the first 3 days, they received 3 capsules (containing 192 mg of chlormethiazole base) 3 times daily, then 2 capsules 3 times daily for 2 days and 3 capsules on the 6th day. Chlormethiazole does not seem to interfere with the hypothalamic releasing factors for pituitary gonadotropins or to affect testicular functions directly.

84. Mendelson, J. H., Ellingboe, J., & Mello, N. K. Ethanol induced alterations in pituitary gonadal hormones in human males. In H. Begleiter (Ed.), *Biological effects of alcohol: Proceedings of the International Symposium on Biological Research in Alcoholism, Zürich, June 1978.* New York: Plenum Press, 1980.

The author's findings of ethanol-induced changes in plasma testosterone, luteinizing hormone, prolactin and gonadotropins, and urinary estrogens in male alcoholics were reviewed. It is suggested that alcohol intoxication alters human male libido and sexual activity is mediated in part by changes in pituitary-gonadal hormones. (RUCAS)

85. Mendelson, J. H., Ellingboe, J., Mello, N. K., & Kuehnle, J. Effects of alcohol on plasma testosterone and luteinizing hormone levels. *Alcoholism: Clinical and Experimental Research,* 1978, *2,* 255–258.

Adult males with no history of alcohol abuse were administered controlled doses of alcohol. Plasma samples were collected every 20 minutes for a period beginning 1 hour before administration and ending 5 hours following alcohol intake. The resulting hormone levels during the ascending, peak, and descending phases of the blood alcohol curve indicated that the major effect of ethanol on plasma testosterone is occurring at a peripheral (testicular) level rather than central (hypothalamic-pituitary) site. The authors postulate that increases in sexual arousal following acute alcohol intake by males are the result of this hormonal activity.

86. Mendelson, J. H., & Mello, N. K. Alkohol, aggression, androgene: alkoholabusus drosselt plasmatestosteronespiegel. [Alcohol, aggression, androgens: Alcohol abuse decreases plasma testosterone levels.] *Sexualmedizin,* 1975, *4,* 646–651.

As is well known, alcohol can promote aggression and perhaps even provoke it. Chronic alcohol abuse impairs the functioning of the reproductive glands and consequently the sexual function. The expression of sexual and aggressive forms of behavior is related to the testosterone content of the blood. The present study on 9 male alcoholics is a contribution toward clarifying the question concerning possible regularities in the interactions between alcohol consumption, aggression, and androgens.

87. Mendelson, J. H., & Mello, N. K. Biologic concomitants of alcoholism. *The New England Journal of Medicine,* 1979, *301,* 912–921.

This review summarizes some recent advances in behavioral and biologic studies of the antecedents and consequences of alcoholism and alcohol abuse. The effects of alcohol on the pituitary and gonadal hormones can lead to testicular atrophy, decreased libido, and impotence. Decrements in sexual performance are associated with alcohol-induced decrements in testosterone levels. It is hypothesized that these problems result from alcohol's interfering with the gonadal steroid function. Alcohol-induced suppression of testosterone is primarily due to ethanol's effect on the testes rather than to an ethanol-mediated effect on the pituitary trophic hormone (luteinizing hormone).

88. Mendelson, J. H., Mello, N. K., & Ellingboe, J. Effects of acute alcohol intake on pituitary-gonadal hormones in normal human males. *The Journal of Pharmacology and Experimental Therapeutics,* 1977, *202,* 676–682.

Plasma luteinizing hormone and testosterone levels were determined in 16 normal adult males during a period of acute alcohol intoxication. Plasma testosterone levels were in the normal range for adult males prior to alcohol administration. Plasma testosterone levels began to fall during the ascending phase of the blood alcohol curve, but plasma luteinizing hormone levels did not change significantly. At peak blood alcohol levels [109 ± 4.6 (S.D.) mg/100 ml], plasma testosterone was significantly depressed, and a significant increase in plasma luteinizing hormone values occurred. During the descending phase of the blood alcohol curve, plasma testosterone levels remained depressed and plasma luteinizing hormone levels decreased toward baseline values. These data indicate that acute alcohol intake produces a suppression of plasma testosterone via peripheral mechanisms that regulate the biosynthesis and/or biotransformation of the steroid. The surge in luteinizing hormone values at peak levels of intoxication are most likely due to stimulation of gonadotropin secretion via ''long loop'' mechanisms associated with low levels of plasma testosterone. (Author)

89. Mendelson, J. H., Mello, N. K., & Ellingboe, J. Effects of alcohol on pituitary-gonadal hormones, sexual function, and aggression in human males. In M. A. Lipton, A. DiMascio, & K. F. Killam, (Eds.), *Psychopharmacology: A generation of progress.* New York: Raven Press, 1978.

Two studies were done examining the interrelationship between alcohol intake and male hormonal homeostasis. The first study examines the effects of ethanol on plasma testosterone levels and estrogen levels in 24-hour urine samples from 8 alcohol addicts studied under research ward conditions. Each subject was used as his own control, and a number of variables that might affect endocrine homeostasis could either be closely monitored or controlled. Hormonal measurements were made prior to, during, and following a prolonged period of chronic high-dosage ethanol intake. The second study looked more precisely at the acute effects of alcohol intake on plasma levels of testosterone and luteinizing hormone in 16 healthy adult males who had no history of alcohol or drug abuse. These subjects also served as their own controls. Hormone levels were determined prior to, during, and following a period of acute alcohol intoxication.

Alcohol-induced decrease in plasma testosterone levels was observed in both studies. Among the alcohol addicts, plasma testosterone levels returned almost to predrinking baseline levels after cessation of alcohol intake. Excretion of urinary estrogens showed no significant change. Discussion includes a review of related endocrine studies and a hypothesis about the implications of these findings for sexual and aggressive behavior in human males.

90. Menendez, C. E. Effects of alcohol on the male reproductive system. In F. S. Messiha (Ed.), *Alcoholism: A perspective* (Vol. 8). Westbury, NY: PJD Publications Ltd., 1980.

Large concentrations of alcohol interfere with the normal function of the male reproductive system. Even before the appearance of liver disease, hypogonadism and feminization may develop. Contributing to feminization of the alcoholic is the altered male-to-female hormone ratio due to the breakdown acceleration of testosterone and the conversion of male hormones to estrogens by alcohol. There is evidence of a suppressive effect of alcohol at both the central and the testicular level in both experimental animals and men, and it may affect the pituitary function as well. Elevated estrogens suppress the male reproductive axis at the hypothalamic and testicular levels. The biochemical mechanisms responsible for these effects of alcohol are unknown. The mainstays of therapy of this syndrome are abstinence from alcohol and adequate psychological and sexual counseling. Replacement doses of testosterone or Vitamin A and zinc may prove beneficial but are still in the experimental stage. (RUCAS)

91. Protici, M., Oprescu, M., Simionescu, L., & Stankusev, T. Nivi no luleotropniya khormon (LTKH) pre muzhe bolni ot alkokholna bolest. [Luteotropic hormone level in male patients with alcoholism.] *Vustreshni Bolesti*, 1977, *16*, 83–85.

The author examined 46 alcoholic males and 10 healthy males aged 20 to 50. Luteotropic hormone levels (LTH) were determined by radioimmunology. A significant decrease in LTH was found in the alcoholics when compared to the healthy controls evidencing the effect of chronic alcoholism on LTH. Alcoholics with and without sexual dysfunction did not differ in LTH levels. The authors presume, therefore, that LTH does not play a role in the sexual dysfunction caused by alcoholism.

92. Rallo, R., Fermoso, J., Ramos, F., Gonzalez-Calvo, V., & Maranon, A. Estudio del eje hipotalamo-hipofisario-gonadal en pacientes alcoholicos cronicos. [A study of hypothalamic-pituitary-gonadal axis in male chronic alcoholism patients.] *Prensa Médica Méxicana*, 1979, *64*, 136–144.

Eleven male chronic alcoholics without cirrhosis but with clinical features of alcoholism were studied. Ten healthy men of similar age served as controls. After follicle-stimulating hormone (FSH), luteinizing hormone (LH), 17β estradiol (E2), and testosterone were determined in basal conditions, and after administration of clomiphene citrate in each case,

basal levels of FSH, LH, and E2 were found to be higher and the testosterone level lower in the alcoholic group. After stimulation, there was no difference in gonadal hormone levels between both groups, suggesting a normal hypothalamic-pituitary axis with an adequate gonadal response. (English abstract was provided as a summary at the beginning of foreign article cited above.) (Author)

93. Rowe, P. H., Racey, P. A., Shenton, J. C., Ellwood, M., & Lehane, J. Effects of acute administration of alcohol and barbiturates on plasma luteinizing hormone and testosterone in man. *Journal of Endocrinology*, 1974, *63*, 50–51.

The acute effects of alcohol and somnific barbiturate doses on plasma luteinizing hormone (LH) and testosterone were studied in healthy nonalcoholic males. Alcohol was found to cause a brief but marked depression in testosterone levels in normally light drinkers and to disturb the daily pattern of LH release. However, alcohol apparently did not alter plasma testosterone in men accustomed to regular heavy drinking. None of the subjects had previously taken barbiturates; administration of 3–6 mg/kg doses had no effect on testosterone levels. No statistically significant changes in LH levels resulted from barbiturate treatment. It is believed that in healthy men alcohol may have a limited importance for the LH-testosterone system.

94. Rubin, E., Lieber, C. S., Altman, K., Gordon, G. G., & Southren, A. L. Prolonged ethanol consumption increases testosterone metabolism in the liver. *Science*, 1976, *191*, 563–564.

Male alcoholics often suffer from features of hypogonadism related to abnormal metabolism of sex steroids. Since the activity of testosterone reductases is rate limiting for testosterone metabolism in the liver, the effect of prolonged ethanol consumption by rats and human volunteers on the activities of these microsomal and cytobolic enzymes was studied. In rats, long-term ethanol ingestion doubled microsomal testosterone reductase activity, a major pathway for testosterone metabolism, while in human volunteers the activity was increased two- to fivefold. These changes may play a role in the altered androgenic activity of the chronic alcoholic. (Author)

95. Simionescu, L., Oprescu, M., Protici, M., & Dimitriu, V. The hormonal pattern in alcoholic disease: I. Luteinizing hormone (LH), follicle-stimulating hormone (FSH) and testosterone. *Romanian Journal of Medicine—Endocrinology*, 1977, *15*, 45–49.

The study included 48 male chronic alcoholics, aged 20 through 50 years, classified in 2 groups according to the presence (22 patients) or absence (26 patients) of clinically evident sexual disorders. Blood samples were collected the first 2–3 days after hospitalization, before any antialcoholic treatment. The control group included 10 adult normal male subjects. By comparison to the control group, the basal level of LH was significantly lower in both groups of alcoholic patients while the FSH level was significantly higher in the group with sexual disorders. The serum levels of testosterone were increased only in the group having sexual disorders. Our data suggest that the feedback regulation of the hypophyseal LH release seems to be impaired by defects in the peripheral metabolization of testosterone. (Author)

96. Sparrow, D., Bosse, R., & Rowe, J. W. The influence of age, alcohol consumption, and body build on gonadal function in men. *Journal of Clinical Endocrinology and Metabolism*, 1980, *51*, 508–512.

No effect of chronic stable alcohol intake level was found on gonadal function, as estimated by testosterone levels and the free testosterone index. Basal plasma levels of testosterone, dihydrotestosterone, estradiol, and gonadotropins and testosterone-binding capacity were measured in healthy, carefully screened, young (31–44 years, N = 44) and old (64–88 years, N = 42) men who were participants in the Normative Aging Study of the Veterans Administration. There was no statistically significant effect of age on testosterone or the free testosterone index. The testosterone binding capacity was higher in the older group ($p < .001$). Of the 2 testosterone products studied, estradiol did not change with age, while dihydrotestosterone was lower in the older group. Follicle-stimulating hormone levels were increased in the older group ($p < .001$). Luteinizing hormone levels were not significantly influenced by age. Estradiol levels were highest in gynandromorphic men and lowest in mesomorphic men. (RUCAS)

97. Van Thiel, D. H. Testicular atrophy and other endocrine changes in alcoholic men. *Medical Aspects of Human Sexuality*, 1976, *10*, 153–154.

The hypothalamic-pituitary-gonadal consequences of alcoholism have been clearly defined over the last several years. The gonadal abnormalities include infertility, sterility, gonadal atrophy, hypoandrogenization, and feminization. The hypothalamic-pituitary abnormalities associated with alcoholism include hyperprolactinemia, lower than expected levels of plasma gonadotropins, and loss of gonadotropin reserve. (Author)

98. Van Thiel, D. H. Alcohol and impotence. *Medical Aspects of Human Sexuality*, 1978, *12*, 11.

In the question and answer section of the journal, a question regarding the relationship between excessive intake of alcohol and impotence is responded to with the observation that alcohol reduces plasma testosterone levels and thereby reduces potency to the extent that testosterone levels contribute to potency.

99. Van Thiel, D. H. An introduction to investigations of metabolic effects of alcohol and alcoholism. In M. Galanter (Ed.), *Currents in Alcoholism* (Vol. 7). New York: Grune & Stratton, 1980.

This chapter reviews 2 broad areas of investigation in metabolic research: (1) the effects of alcohol metabolism upon endocrine function and (2) the effects of alcohol upon brain growth and development. Mention is made of the inhibitory effects of alcohol on hypothalamic-pituitary function and the toxic effect on the gonads.

100. Van Thiel, D. H., Gavaler, J. S., Eagon, P. K., & Lester, R. Effect of alcohol on gonadal function. *Drug and Alcohol Dependence*, 1980, *6*, 41–42. (Abstract of paper presented at the Fifth Biennial International Symposium on Alcoholism, Cardiff, Wales, June 1980.)

Hypogonadism, seen commonly in 70–80% of male alcoholics, is manifested in decreased libido or impotence and testicular atrophy with a marked loss of normal germ cells and an increase of grossly abnormal germ cells. Long-term alcoholics also are hyperestrogenized. Evidence suggests that sexual dysfunction is an early symptom in alcohol-abusing men and animals and that it can occur without histologic liver disease. Alcohol and acetaldehyde are testicular toxins. Testosterone concentrations fall transiently in normal men after alcohol ingestion. Alcohol metabolism may also shift the balance between NAD and NADH and suppress hypothalamic-pituitary function. Other data suggest that alcohol produces a primary hypogonadism and induces a central hypothalamic-pituitary defect in gonadotropin secretion, even in the absence of liver cirrhosis. (RUCAS)

101. Van Thiel, D. H., & Lester, R. Further evidence for hypothalamic-pituitary dysfunction in alcoholic men. *Alcoholism: Clinical and Experimental Research*, 1978, *2*, 265–270.

Reduced plasma levels of testosterone and a high frequency of azoospermia have frequently been reported in alcoholic men. Despite the high grade of gonadal failure present, plasma gonadotropins have ranged from normal to only moderately increased. This has been interpreted as suggesting that a central hypothalamic-pituitary defect also might exist in these men. Clomiphene stimulation studies have been consistent with the hypothesis of a central defect. The present work consists of studies utilizing luteinizing hormone-releasing factor and thyrotropin-releasing factor in an effort to examine the hypothesis of whether this central defect exists and, if so, whether at an anatomic, hypothalamic, or pituitary level. (Author)

102. Wright, J. W., Fry, D. E., Merry, J., & Marks, V. Abnormal hypothalamic-pituitary-gonadal function in chronic alcoholics. *British Journal of Addictions*, 1976, *71*, 211–215.

Hypothalamic-pituitary-gonadal function was investigated in a group of 13 actively drinking alcoholic men, and it was found that in a high proportion (46%) of the patients basal plasma luteinizing hormone (LH) levels were elevated. Stimulation with a luteinizing hormone releasing factor resulted in a rise in plasma LH in all subjects. Plasma levels of 17β-hydroxyandrogens were not significantly different in the alcoholic patients and control subjects of comparable age, although intragroup variation was especially wide in the alcoholic group. Several mechanisms are suggested to explain the imbalance in sex steroids which is frequently seen in alcoholic persons. Liver damage did not appear to explain the biochemical findings of this study. (NCALI)

103. Ylikahri, R., Huttunen, M., Harkonen, M., & Adlercreutz, H. Hangover and testosterone. *British Medical Journal*, 1974, *2*, 445.

Ten healthy male students aged 19 to 25 were administered alcohol (1.5 g/kg as a 20% aqueous solution) at a constant rate for 3 hours from 6 P.M. to 9 P.M. By the next morning all the subjects had a more or less severe hangover. Blood samples for determining levels of luteinizing hormone and testosterone were taken at the start of drinking and at 4, 8, 12, 15, and 20 hours afterwards. During acute intoxication there were no changes in plasma testosterone concentrations. During hangover, 12–20 hours after the start of drinking, testosterone was decreased. Decrease seemed to correlate with intensity of the hangover. Plasma LH increased slightly during hangover. This study offers evidence that alcohol can alter sex hormone metabolism without causing liver damage.

104. Ylikahri, R. H., Huttunen, M., Harkonen, M., Seuderling, U., Onikki, S., Karonen, S. L., & Adlercreutz, H. Low plasma testosterone values in men during hangover. *Journal of Steroid Biochemistry*, *1974, 5*, 655–658.

Plasma testosterone, estradiol, and luteinizing hormone concentrations were measured by radioimmunoassay in healthy volunteers who, after fasting for 10 hours, consumed 1.5 grams of ethanol per kilogram of body weight. Of this group, 5 suffered from severe hangover while another 5 had essentially no hangover. Ten to 20 hours after drinking, the testosterone concentrations were significantly decreased in all subjects, but in the 5 subjects with severe hangover the decrease was more pronounced. Estradiol values decreased during the hangover period but were normal at the time of acute intoxication, whereas estrone values in the few cases determined showed a tendency to increase during acute intoxication. A compensatory increase in the plasma concentration of luteinizing hormone was found in all subjects. (Author)

2. Alcoholic Cirrhosis and Sexual Behavior

a. Both Sexes

105. Gastineau, C. F. Alcohol and the endocrine system. In P. Avogaro, C. R. Sirtori, & E. Tremoli (Eds.), *Metabolic Effects of Alcohol: Proceedings of the International Symposium on Metabolic Effects of Alcohol held in Milan (Italy) on June 18-21, 1979.* New York: Elsevier, 1979.

The authors summarize what is known about alcohol's effect on the endocrine system. The complexities and inconsistencies of current knowledge are highlighted. Disturbances in endocrine function, particularly sex hormone metabolism, are found with or without the presence of liver disease. A unifying theory to explain and predict the endocrine effects of alcohol is needed.

106. Gordon, G. G., Vittek, J., Ho, R., Rosenthal, W. S., Southren, A. L., & Lieber, C. S. Effect of chronic alcohol use on hepatic testosterone 5α-A-ring reductase in the baboon and in the human being. *Gastroenterology*, 1979, *77*, 110–114.

Testosterone 5α-A-ring reductase (HTAR) activity was measured in liver biopsies from 16 female baboons pair-fed liquid diets containing 50% of calories as alcohol or additional carbohydrate for 1–6 years. Hepatic histology of the alcohol-fed baboons ranged from normal to fully developed cirrhosis. Their HTAR activity was significantly decreased whether expressed in relation to soluble protein, to DNA, or to wet tissue weight ($p < .05$ or $.01$). Further, HTAR activity was significantly lower in aspiration liver biopsies from 14 hospitalized patients (aged 29–63; 3 women) with active cirrhosis or alcoholic hepatitis than in 11 healthy subjects (2 women) of similar age distribution ($p < .001$). No correlation was found between hepatic histology and HTAR levels in either the baboon or human populations with alcoholic liver disease, suggesting that the changes in enzyme activity were an effect of alcohol rather than of liver disease per se. (RUCAS)

107. Greene, L. W., & Hollander, C. S. Sex and alcohol: The effects of alcohol on the hypothalamic-pituitary-gonadal axis. *Alcoholism: Clinical and Experimental Research*, 1980, *4*, 1–5.

Hypogonadism (accompanied by impotence, testicular atrophy, and sterility) and feminization (with the loss of the male pattern of secondary sex hair, development of gynecomastia, and vascular changes) is a prominent clinical syndrome in the male alcoholic. It is, therefore, not surprising that the preponderance of work on the endocrine effects of alcohol has focused on the hypothalamic-pituitary-gonadal axis. In contrast, the female alcoholic syndromes of menstrual abnormalities, anovulation, signs of estrogen deprivation in the uterus and fallopian tubes, and placental malfunction have only recently been documented. The authors attempt to place these clinical findings in perspective, review research on the hypothalamic-pituitary-gonadal system, identify those areas in which a consensus has developed, and pinpoint new areas for further exploration. (Author)

108. Kayusheva, I. V. Alkogolizm i endokrinnaya sistema. [Alcoholism and the endocrine system.] *Sovetskaia Meditsina* (Moskva), 1979, *7*, 87–91.

The literature on the effect of alcoholism on the endocrine system is reviewed. Particular attention is paid to the effect of alcoholism on the hypothalamus, pituitary, and adrenal cortex. Other glands discussed are the thyroid, the testes and ovaries, the pancreas, and the thymus. (RUCAS)

109. Lloyd, C. W., & Williams, R. H. Endocrine changes associated with Laennec's cirrhosis of the liver. *American Journal of Medicine*, 1948, *4*, 315–330.

Seventy-one patients with cirrhosis of the liver were studied to investigate the role of the liver in steroid metabolism and endocrine disturbances accompanying cirrhosis. Fifty-five male and 16 female patients were studied. Patients were categorized by severity of liver disease. Severity of endocrine disturbances, manifested by decreased libido, decrease in axillary hair, testicular atrophy and gynecomastia in males, and menstrual irregularities and atrophy of the breasts in women, all increased with degree of liver pathology. Among males, decrease in libido was one of the earliest symptoms noted, followed by loss of potency. Of the 2 patients with mild cirrhosis, one reported slight, but noticeable decrease in libido with no change in potency. Five of the 7 cases with moderate cirrhosis reported decrease in libido with 2 reporting erectile dysfunction as well. Forty-six males had severe cirrhosis; 31 of these showed definitely decreased libido and potency. Data on females' change in libido were not broken down by severity of cirrhosis. The article simply reports that there is a decrease.

110. Miyazaki, T., & Araki, Y. [Abnormal steroid hormone metabolism during administration of various drugs.] *Nippon Rinsho* [Japanese Journal of Clinical Medicine], 1979, *37*, 1283–1288.

111. Rallo, R., Fermoso, J., Escorial, C., Ergueta, P., Blanco, J., & Maranon, A. Fisiopatologia del eje hipotalamo-hipofisario-gonadal en el alcoholismo cronico y en la cirrosis hepatica. [Physiopathology of the hypothalamic-hypophyseal-gonadal axis in chronic alcoholism and liver cirrhosis: Review and update.] *Prensa Médica Méxicana*, 1979, *64*, 129–135.

112. Scheig, R. Changes in sexual performance due to liver disease. *Medical Aspects of Human Sexuality*, 1975, *9*, 67–79.

Most patients with chronic liver disease suffer from problems in sexual performance, but very few complain about it. Young women are usually upset about their appearance, their lack of menses, and the fact that they probably will bear no children. Males with chronic liver disease and organic impotency usually do not benefit from medical or psychologic therapy. Wives, however, are usually helped by rather intensive counseling. Those patients with minimal liver disease, and especially those whose problems are primarily due to excessive alcohol intake, can often be helped greatly if they can be persuaded to cease their alcohol consumption and seek appropriate counselling for their sexual maladjustments. Three case histories are presented to illustrate the effects. (Author)

113. Stiasna, I., Grabowska-Hibner, J., & Szukalski, B. Biochemiczne aspekty alkoholizmu: II. Wplyw etanolu na przemiany bialek i sterydow. [Biochemical aspects of alcoholism: II. Influence of ethanol on the turnover of steroids and proteins.] *Postepy Higieny i Medycyny Doswiadczalnej*, 1979, *33*, 325–343.

Review of current literature concerning the effect of ethanol on the metabolism of proteins and steroid hormones is presented. (English abstract and English title were provided as a summary at the end of foreign article cited above.) (Author)

114. Stocks, A. E., & Powell, L. W. Pituitary function in idiopathic haemochromatosis and cirrhosis of the liver. *The Lancet*, 1972, *2*, 298–300.

Of 22 patients with liver cirrhosis (8 women), 16 were alcoholics. Decreased sexual function was present in 47% of the patients (among them only 1 woman). Testicular atrophy was found in 10 men; their plasma levels of the luteinizing hormone were normal. Other indices of gonadal hypofunction were present only in men. These findings are probably the result of ineffective estrogen metabolism by the cirrhotic liver.

115. Valimaki, M., & Ylikahri, R. Alcohol and sex hormones. *Scandinavian Journal of Clinical and Laboratory Investigation*, 1981, *41*, 99–105.

Alcohol induces hypoandrogenization through its direct effects on the testes and also by interrupting the pituitary gonadotropin secretion. Alcohol-induced hepatic changes also contribute to hypoandrogenization by stimulating testosterone catabolism. Measurements of the hormone concentrations in plasma suggest that hyperestrogenization of chronic male alcoholics is mainly due to increased plasma concentration of estrone. Alcohol increases the secretion of the precursors of estrone from the adrenal cortex. The conversion of these precursors to estrone is increased in alcoholics. Alcohol induces sexual dysfunction in women also, but the mechanisms are unknown. (RUCAS)

116. Ylikahri, R. Alkoholin endokrinologiset vaikutukset. [The endocrine effects of alcohol.] *Duodecim*, 1979, *95*, 410–419.

117. Ylikahri, R. H., Huttunen, M. O., & Härkönen, M. Hormonal changes during alcohol intoxication and withdrawal. *Pharmacology, Biochemistry & Behavior*, 1980, *13*, (Supplement 1), 134–137.

The endocrine effects of alcohol are briefly reviewed. Alcohol enhances glucose-induced insulin secretion and may thus cause reactive hypoglycemia. However, inappropriate insulin secretion is not the reason for alcohol-induced hypoglycemia in fasted subjects. The direct effects of alcohol on thyroid function in humans are small, although alcoholics often have low concentrations of thyroid hormones in their plasma because of liver damage. Alcohol increases cortisol secretion from adrenal cortex either by increasing ACTH secretion or, more probably, by directly stimulating the adrenals. Alcohol also increases aldosterone secretion. The production of epinephrine and norepinephrine by the adrenal medulla is increased during alcohol intoxication and withdrawal. Plasma testosterone concentration is decreased during hangover and during alcohol withdrawal. The decrease is due to direct effects of alcohol on the testes, because plasma LH concentration is increased simultaneously. Alcohol has no significant effect on the LRH-induced secretion of LH. Plasma growth hormone concentration is decreased during alcohol intoxication and increased during hangover. TRH-induced secretion of prolactin is increased during alcohol intoxication and inhibited during hangover and withdrawal. The last finding suggests that there is dopaminergic overactivity in hypothalamus during alcohol withdrawal. (Author)

b. Females

118. Hugues, J. N., Perret, G., Adessi, G., Coste, T., & Modigliani, E. Effects of chronic alcoholism on the pituitary-gonadal function of women during menopausal transition and in the post menopausal period. *Biomedicine*, 1978, *29*, 279–283.

The hypothalamic-pituitary-gonadal function was evaluated in 11 chronically alcoholic menopausal women by measurement of basal serum estradiol, FSH, LH, and prolactin, followed by LHRH-TRH test and administration of clomiphene citrate. All patients had hepatic damage, fibrosteatosis, or cirrhosis. Two subgroups, postmenopausal and menopausal transition, have been isolated according to urinary and serum estrogen levels. Seven patients with urinary estrogen output less than $14 \mu g/24$ hours and plasma estradiol less than 40 pg/ml were considered postmenopausal women. Basal values of FSH and LH and their response to LHRH did not differ from that observed in normal menopausal women. Clomiphene citrate induced a significant suppression of FSH and LH blood levels. Four women with urinary estrogen output greater than $14 \mu g/24$ hours and plasma estradiol greater than 40 pg/ml were considered in menopausal transition. Their basal and post LHRH-FSH blood levels were lower than in the control group. These results suggest a normal hypothalamic-pituitary-gonadal axis at least in postmenopausal alcoholic women. (Author)

c. Males

119. Baker, H. W. G., Burger, H. G., de Kretser, D. M., Dulmanis, A., Hudson, B., O'Connor, S., Paulsen, C. A., Purcell, N., Rennie, G. C., Seah, C. S., Taft, H. P., & Wang, C. A study of the endocrine manifestations of hepatic cirrhosis. *Quarterly Journal of Medicine*, 1976, *45*, 145–178.

The clinical features and hormonal abnormalities were surveyed in 117 men with cirrhosis of the liver. Compared with healthy men of similar ages, the patients had significantly lower metabolic clearance rates, plasma production rates, and total and free levels of testosterone, reduced testosterone responses to human chorionic gonadotropin stimulation, higher estradiol, luteinizing hormone, and follicle-stimulating hormone levels, and higher binding capacities of sex-steroid-binding globulin. The peripheral conversion of testosterone to estradiol was also found to be significantly increased. However, the metabolic clearance and plasma production rates of estradiol were not significantly different from those of healthy men. Patients who were severely ill with liver failure and one with haemochromatosis had low levels of luteinizing hormone and follicle-stimulating hormone and subnormal responses to clomiphene and luteinizing hormone-releasing hormone. Higher plasma estradiol levels were found in patients with gynecomastia and spider naevi than in those without these signs. However, the clinical features of androgen deficiency—that is, testicular atrophy, impotence, and loss of secondary sex hair—were only poorly related to the low testosterone levels, and production rates; and longitudinal studies indicated that the hormonal levels, endocrine features, and severity of the liver disease could change independently. (Author)

120. Bjork, J. T., Varma, R. R., & Borkowf, H. I. Clomiphene citrate therapy in a patient with Laennec's cirrhosis. *Gastroenterology*, 1977, *72*, 1308–1311.

Clomiphene citrate therapy was initiated in a male with Laennec's cirrhosis complicated by gynecomastia, testicular atrophy, impotence, and loss of libido. The patient had abstained from alcohol and had stable hepatic function tests for 1 year before starting therapy. Luteinizing hormone and endogenous testosterone levels were maximally elevated with low dose therapy (50 mg/day). Follicle-stimulating hormone was maximally elevated with a dose of 100 mg/day and the elevation of total estrogen levels was not affected by increasing the dose. During treatment, increase in testicular size was noted with resolution of impotence and improvement of libido, which continued for 6 months after cessation of therapy. Gynecomastia remained unchanged despite the increased serum testosterone. Serum prolactin was normal before and after the clomiphene citrate. Semen initially unobtainable was analyzed after completion of therapy. The patient relapsed 8 months after the course of clomiphene citrate therapy. (Author)

121. Cedard, L., Mosse, A., & Klotz, H. P. Les oestrogènes plasmatiques dans les gynécomasties et les hépatopathies. [Plasmatic oestrogens in gynecomastias and hepatopathies.] *Annales d'Endocrinologie*, 1970, *31*, 453–458.

The frequent occurrence of endocrine disorders in cirrhoses has led us to study estrogens in peripheral plasma in chronic hepatopathies and gynecomastias of various origins. The fractionated fluorometric measurement of total estrogens after hydrolysis allowed us to show in a very great number of patients a hyper-estrogenemia and, in cases of gynecomastia, a very characteristic rise in the estradiol-estrone ratio. It is, therefore, possible to attribute responsibility for the clinical symptoms of hyperestrogeny to the excess of estradiol in the peripheral venous blood. (English abstract and English title were provided as a summary at the beginning of foreign article cited above.) (Author)

122. Chopra, I. J., Tulchinsky, D., & Greenway, F. L. Estrogen-androgen imbalance in hepatic cirrhosis: Studies in 13 male patients. *Annals of Internal Medicine*, 1973, *79*, 198–203.

Serum concentrations of testosterone, dihydrotestosterone, estradiol-17β (E_2), and gonadotropins were studied in 13 male patients with hepatic cirrhosis. The mean serum total and unbound testosterone concentrations were significantly lower in the cirrhotic patients than in normal men. Serum dihydrotestosterone levels were also subnormal in 5 of 6 patients studied. On the other hand, the mean serum total and unbound E_2 concentrations were significantly higher in patients with cirrhosis than in normal men. The most consistent abnormality and the one uniformly present was a supranormal E_2 to testosterone ratio, as calculated from serum concentration of total or unbound steroids. These findings suggest that changes in the relative balance between circulating estrogen and androgen may play some part in the pathogenesis of gynecomastia in hepatic cirrhosis. The mean serum luteinizing hormone concentration was elevated in patients with cirrhosis, whereas that of follicle-stimulating hormone did not differ from normal. (Author)

123. Distiller, L. A., Sagel, J., Dubowitz, B., Kay, G., Carr, P. J., Katz, M., & Kew, M. C. Pituitary-gonadal function in men with alcoholic cirrhosis of the liver. *Hormone Metabolism Research*, 1976, *8*, 461–465.

Fourteen adult males with alcoholic cirrhosis were studied. Gonadotropin responses to luteinizing hormone-releasing hormone (LRH) and testosterone (T) responses to human chorionic gonadtropin (HCG) were determined and basal 17β-estradiol (E$_2$) levels were measured in each case. The mean basal luteinizing hormone (LH) and follicle-stimulating hormone (FSH) levels and the mean LH and FSH responses to LRH were not significantly different from a group of age-matched male controls. However, the 5 men with testicular atrophy all had an elevated basal FSH level and an exaggerated FSH response to LRH. The mean serum T of the cirrhotic men was significantly different. However, the mean E$_2$ level in the 8 patients with gynecomastia was significantly higher than in those without gynecomastia. All patients had a T response to HCG, including those 5 with low basal T levels. A significant negative correlation was found between the maximum rise in T after HCG ($\triangle$T) and the maximum LH response to LRH ($\triangle$LH), suggesting a mediating effect of T reserve on the LH response to LRH. These findings tend to exclude a suppressive effect of alcohol on the pituitary gland as a cause for the hypogonadism found in men with alcoholic cirrhosis. Furthermore, the evidence of some testicular T reserve despite low basal T levels, and the presence of normal basal LH levels, suggests that the low T production is not primarily due to Leydig cell dysfunction. (Author)

124. Farnsworth, W. E., Cavanaugh, A. H., Brown, J. R., Alvarez, I., & Lewandowski, L. M. Factors underlying infertility in the alcoholic. *Archives of Andrology*, 1978, *1*, 193–195.

In an effort to identify the factor(s) contributing to loss in sexual competence in alcoholics, a pilot study was made of the interrelationships of hepatic disease, plasma hormone levels, and impotence in 35 male patients in an alcohol unit. Contrary to previous reports, impotence was not a direct concomitant of hepatic disease, elevated sex-hormone-binding globulin capacity, or hyperestrinism. The most significant aberration found was a nearly 30% lower mean free testosterone concentration which appeared to be secondary to a mean total testosterone concentration 20% below that of the subjects with normal sexual function. We conclude from this that impotence results from testicular secretion impaired by the action of alcohol or its metabolite, acetaldehyde. (Author)

125. Galvão-Teles, A., Anderson, D. C., Burke, C. W., Marshall, J. C., Corker, C. S., Brown, R. L., & Clark, M. L. Biologically active androgens and oestradiol in men with chronic liver disease. *The Lancet*, 1973, *1*, 173–177.

Twenty-five men with chronic liver disease were studied. The plasma levels of unbound (biologically active) 17β-hydroxyandrogens (17-OHA), principally testosterone, were significantly lower in them than in controls (means 99 and 160 pg/ml, respectively). This fall was most striking in the patients with alcoholic cirrhosis (mean 68 pg/ml). Serum-luteinizing-hormone (LH) was high (mean of 2.35 mU/ml in controls; 3.7 mU/ml in patients). Unbound-plasma-estradiol levels were normal. Plasma sex-hormone-binding globulin (SHBG) concentrations were raised twofold although the albumin levels were reduced. It is suggested that in men with chronic liver disease increased hepatic SHBG production causes the fall in unbound-plasma-17-OHA levels and that the hypothalamus responds to this by stimulating increased LH production. Apparently this does not increase Leydig cell production of testosterone enough to return the unbound level to normal. The normal unbound estradiol levels may be maintained because the effect of the fall in plasma-albumin on estradiol-binding cancels out the opposite effect of a rise in SHBG. It is suggested that the combination of normal unbound-plasma-estradiol and reduced unbound androgen levels may lead to gynecomastia and clinical evidence of hypogonadism in chronic liver disease. The greater reduction in unbound-plasma-17-OHA in alcoholic cirrhosis may be a factor responsible for the higher frequency of gynecomastia and hypogonadism in this form of liver disease. (Author)

126. Gluud, C., Hardt, F., Juhl, E., Bennett, P., & Johnsen, S. G. Endocrine aspects of liver disease. *British Medical Journal*, 1980, *280*, 1452.

In response to a review article concluding that there is no evidence that testosterone treatment of cirrhosis is beneficial, the authors point out studies demonstrating the positive effects of such treatment on complications, sexual impotence, and survival. Duration of treatment must be longer than one month to obtain any effect. The safety of long-term treatment may depend on the form of testosterone used in treatment, for there are no reports of side effects from genuine testosterone. Controlled studies using genuine testosterone in treatment of men with alcoholic liver disease are needed to establish effects and side effects.

127. Gordon, G. G., Olivo, J., Rafii, F., & Southren, A. L. Conversion of androgens to estrogens in cirrhosis of the liver. *Journal of Clinical Endocrinology and Metabolism*, 1975, *40*, 1018–1026.

The contribution, by peripheral conversion, of androstenedione and testosterone to the circulating estrogens was determined in men with cirrhosis of the liver. The conversion ratio of androstenedione to estrone, estradiol, and testosterone and the conversion ratio of testosterone to estrone (but not estradiol) and androstenedione were significantly increased. The plasma concentrations of androstenedione and testosterone were increased and decreased respectively, the mean plasma concentration of androstenedione being similar to that found in normal women. The metabolic clearance rate of androstenedione was not altered in cirrhosis although the metabolic clearance rate of testosterone was decreased. The production rate of androstenedione was elevated while that of testosterone was reduced. The instantaneous contribution of plasma androstenedione to estrone and estradiol was increased in cirrhosis as was the contribution of testosterone to estrone (but not to estradiol). Thus the increased estradiol levels in cirrhosis result, in large part, from increased peripheral conversion from the androgens. The percent contribution of plasma testosterone to plasma androstenedione was decreased although the absolute amount derived by conversion was normal. The percent contribution of plasma androstenedione to plasma testosterone was increased sevenfold in cirrhosis. The fraction of the daily androstenedione production derived from the plasma testosterone pool was not significantly altered. However, a significant fraction of the daily production rate of testosterone was derived from androstenedione. Thus, 15% of the circulating testosterone is not secreted but is derived by peripheral conversion from androstenedione. Normal levels of gonadotropins were found in cirrhosis. (Author)

128. Gordon, G. G., Vittek, J., Weinstein, B., Southren, A. L., & Lieber, C. S. Acute and chronic effects of alcohol on steroid hormones with emphasis on the metabolism of androgens and estrogens. In P. Avogaro, C. R. Sirtori, & E. Tremoli (Eds.), *Metabolic Effects of Alcohol: Proceedings of the International Symposium on Metabolic Effects of Alcohol held in Milan (Italy) on June 18-21, 1979.* New York: Elsevier, 1979.

This review focuses primarily on the effect of alcohol on sex hormone metabolism. Evidence exists for a direct hypothalamic-pituitary effect decreasing plasma testosterone during acute and chronic exposure to alcohol. In men and women with alcoholic liver disease, alcohol appears to influence plasma testosterone levels via gonadal suppressive effects and perturbations in peripheral steroid metabolism as well.

129. Hormones trip cirrhotic sex changes. *Medical World News*, December 7, 1973, p. 24.

An imbalance of the pituitary-gonadal system was shown to be the cause of male sexual dysfunction linked with alcoholic cirrhosis in an experimental study. The study was conducted by David H. Van Thiel and Roger Lester of the University of Pittsburgh School of Medicine. The "feminization" was attributed to low levels of pituitary hormones (FSH and LH) and of gonadal hormone (testosterone), and to the sluggish response of both hormones to exogenous stimulation. Accordingly, the theory of the etiological role of liver dysfunction (i.e., the inability of the liver to remove excess steroidal estrogen from the body) is discounted. The specific findings of this study and the prognosis for patients with cirrhosis-related sexual problems are discussed.

130. Kent, J. R., Scaramuzzi, R. J., Lauwers, W., Parlow, A. F., Hill, M., Penardi, R., & Hilliard, J. Plasma testosterone, estradiol, and gonadotrophins in hepatic insufficiency. *Gastroenterology*, 1973, *64*, 111–115.

The pituitary-gonadal axis was evaluated in 22 male patients with hepatic insufficiency, utilizing measurements of serum estradiol, testosterone (T), follicle-stimulating hormone, and

luteinizing hormone. In these patients, only levels of T were significantly different from those obtained in normal men (3.9 ng/ml in patients versus 5.2 ng/ml in normal subjects, P<0.05). Levels of follicle-stimulating hormone and luteinizing hormone were normal even in patients with markedly low serum T. In none of the patients with low serum T were gonadotropins elevated to levels expected in primary testicular failure. The pathophysiology of hypogonadism in this disease may be more complicated than previous studies have indicated. (Author)

131. Kley, H. K., Nieschlag, E., Wiegelmann, W., Solbach, H. G., & Krüskemper, H. L. Steroid hormones and their binding in plasma of male patients with fatty liver, chronic hepatitis and liver cirrhosis. *Acta Endocrinologica*, 1975, *79*, 275–285.

Estrone (E1), estradiol (E2), testosterone (T), androstenedione (A), and cortisol (F), as well as LH and the percentage of binding of E1, E2, T, and F in plasma, were measured and compared in normal young and old male subjects and in male patients with fatty liver, chronic hepatitis, and cirrhosis of the liver. The alterations seen were most marked in the cirrhotic patients, but were partially also found in patients with fatty liver and in normal old subjects: a definite increase in E1, a smaller increase in E2, a decrease in T, and a rise in LH. F remained unchanged. The ratios of E2/T and E1/T were higher in cirrhotic patients than in healthy young subjects. As the percentage of bound T in plasma rose, the estrogen/androgen imbalance was greater in patients with liver disease and in old subjects than the ratio of total hormone plasma concentration indicates. The biological relevance of the extremely high E1 plasma concentrations in patients with cirrhosis of the liver is not known. It is suggested that the combination of elevated E1 and E2 and reduced T, which is strongly bound by increased sex-hormone-binding globulin (SHBG) may be responsible for gynecomastia and hypogonadism in chronic liver diseases. As similar alterations of steroid plasma concentrations and their binding to plasma proteins are found both in patients with liver disease and in old men, these changes may be caused by the same mechanism: namely an altered liver function. (Author)

132. Kley, H. K., Strohmeyer, G., & Krüskemper, H. L. Effect of testosterone application on hormone concentrations of androgens and estrogens in male patients with cirrhosis of the liver. *Gastroenterology*, 1979, *76*, 235–241.

The effect of testosterone enanthate administration was studied in 20 male patients with cirrhosis of the liver and 8 normal controls by the measurement of testosterone (T), androstenedione (A), estrone (E1), and estradiol (E2), as well as of free T and free E2 in the plasma. The patient group was divided into 3 categories (I–III) according to clinical symptoms. Under basal conditions, T was decreased in the plasma, whereas A, E1, and E2 were mainly increased in the patients of groups II and III (patients with gynecomastia and those with gynecomastia and ascites). Minimal hormonal changes were observed in patients without gynecomastia (group I). The balance between sexual hormones, which in cirrhosis of the liver is greatly enhanced in favor of the estrogens, was nearly "normalized" after T-administration. It is concluded that the increased conversion of androgens to estrogens leads to higher estrogen plasma values after exogenous T-administration. Nevertheless, because of the greatly elevated T-values, the imbalance between sexual hormones, which sometimes has been considered to be responsible for signs of increased estrogenic activity in the patients, is nearly normalized. (Author)

133. Lester, R., Van Thiel, D. H., Eagon, P. K., Imhoff, A. F., & Fisher, S. E. Hypothesis concerning the effects of dietary nonsteroidal estrogen on the feminization of male alcoholics. In T.-K. Li, S. Schenker, & L. Lumeng (Eds.), *Alcohol and nutrition: Proceedings of a workshop, September 26-27, 1977,* Indianapolis, Indiana. (NIAAA Research Monograph No. 2, DHEW Publication No. ADM 79–780.) Washington, DC: U.S. Government Printing Office, 1979.)

It is difficult to explain the marked hyperestrogenization of alcoholic men in terms of measureable levels of plasma steroidal estrogen. It is possible that the observed hyperestrogenization is due to the accumulation of dietary nonsteroidal estrogen as the result of liver disease. One means to approach this problem is through the use of a protein-binding assay, using the discriminatory characteristics of the binding proteins in male and female rat liver cytosol. Studies are now in progress to explore this hypothesis. (Author)

134. Lindholm, J., Fabricius-Bjerre, N., Bahnsen, M., Boiesen, P., Bangstrup, L., Lau Pedersen, M., & Hagen, C. Pituitary-testicular function in patients with chronic alcoholism. *European Journal of Clinical Investigation,* 1978, *8,* 269–272.

Testis and liver histology, and pituitary-testicular function were studied in 30 chronic alcoholics. Severe reduction of spermatogenesis was found in 30% and in these patients serum follicle-stimulating hormone and prolactin concentrations were significantly higher. There was no correlation between abnormalities in the liver and testis. The serum testosterone was normal in most cases. Sexual dysfunction and testicular atrophy occurred in more than half of the patients and were not related to liver disease. Testicular disorder in chronic alcoholism may be independent of liver disease. (Author)

135. McClain, C. J., Van Thiel, D. H., Parker, S., Badzin, L. K., & Gilbert, H. Alterations in zinc, Vitamin A, and retinol-binding protein in chronic alcoholics: A possible mechanism for night blindness and hypogonadism. *Alcoholism: Clinical and Experimental Research,* 1979, *3,* 135–141.

Deficiencies in zinc and Vitamin A may play a role in the night blindness and hypogonadism of some chronic alcoholics; abstinence and zinc and Vitamin A therapy may be of some benefit in these processes. (Author)

136. Merry, J. Endocrine response to ethanol: A review of research and clinical studies. *International Journal of Mental Health,* 1976, *5,* 16–28.

This review includes studies of the effects of alcohol on the hypothalamic-pituitary-adrenal system, the sympathetic-adrenal medullary system, insulin and glucagon metabolism, thyroid, and gonads. Signs of feminization, indicating disruption of sex steroid metabolism, are common among alcoholics. Reduced plasma testosterone was observed in 3 of the 5 studies reviewed. Two possible explanations have been hypothesized: (1) that changes in steroid metabolism is the result of liver damage, and (2) that hypogonadism may be due to hypothalamic-pituitary insufficiency. One study reported an absence of feminization among noncirrhotic alcoholics. However, luteinizing hormone was elevated while plasma androgens were normal. Liver damage did not appear to explain the biochemical findings.

137. Mowat, N. A. G., Edwards, C. R. W., Fisher, R., McNeilly, A. S., Green, J. R. B., & Dawson, A. M. Hypothalamic-pituitary gonadal function in men with cirrhosis of the liver. *Gut,* 1976, *17,* 345–350.

Hypothalamic-pituitary-gonadal function was studied in 37 cirrhotic males, 25 of whom were alcoholic. All had significantly reduced free testosterone concentrations and reduced or absent spermatogenesis. Basal levels of luteinizing hormone (LH) and follicle-stimulating hormone (FSH) were normal in nearly all patients, suggesting impaired function of the hypothalamic-pituitary-gonadal axis. In 14 cirrhotic men, 7 of whom had gynecomastia, the ability of the pituitary to secrete LH and FSH in response to exogenous gonadotropin releasing-hormone (LH/FSH-RH) was assessed. A normal LH response to the LH/FSH-RH was obtained in patients without gynecomastia. An exaggerated LH response was found in 4 of 7 with gynecomastia, suggesting Leydig cell failure. The Leydig cell response to exogenous gonadotropin in 8 consecutive cirrhotic patients was probably abnormal but difficult to interpret as all but one were within conventionally accepted limits of normality. The patients without gynecomastia gave a normal or minimally exaggerated FSH response to LH/FSH-RH. Six of 7 with gynecomastia gave a markedly exaggerated response suggesting failure of spermatogenesis, and all tested were either azoospermic or oligospermic. The single patient with a normal FSH response had a normal sperm count. The pituitary cells can therefore respond to LH/FSH-RH and the Leydig cells of the testes show some response to exogenous gonadotropin. (Author)

138. Munjack, D. J. Sex and drugs. *Clinical Toxicology,* 1979, *15,* 75–89.

The neurological and endocrinological effects of alcohol and alcoholism on sex functions are described. As a central depressant, alcohol slows down general responses and lessens acute sensory sensitivity, and peripheral neuropathy associated with alcoholism can contribute to organic sex dysfunctions by cutting down on sensory input and decreasing sexual stimulation. The endocrinological effects include an increase in free plasma estradiol levels in men with advanced Laennec's cirrhosis; increased plasma estrone and prolactin levels (which may lead to gynecomastia and feminization); reduced plasma androgen levels, and more specifically, reduced plasma concentrations resulting from toxicity to Leydig cells and the faster conversion of androgens to estrogens by the cirrhotic liver; abnormal seminal fluid characteristics and altered testicular histology in cirrhotics; and reduction of hypothalamic or pituitary gonadotropin secretions. A possible sequence of events is outlined and the long-term effects of alcohol-induced sexual impotence are discussed, with some attention on alcoholism and marital problems. (RUCAS)

139. Silvestrini, R. La reviviscenza mammaria nell'uomo affetto da cirrosi del Laennec. [Gynecomastia in men with Laennec's cirrhosis.] *La Riforma Medica,* 1926, *142,* 701–704.

140. Southren, A. L., & Gordon, G. G. Effects of alcohol and alcoholic cirrhosis on sex hormone metabolism. *Fertility and Sexuality,* 1976, *27,* 202. (Abstract of paper presented at the 32nd Annual Meeting of the American Fertility Society, Las Vegas, April 1976.)

It is well-known that male patients with alcoholic liver disease frequently develop hypogonadism and feminization. The mechanism of these abnormalities has been clarified to some extent by the observation that alcoholic cirrhosis is associated with a decrease and increase, respectively, in the plasma production rates of testosterone and the estrogens (estradiol and estrone). The major source of the estrogens was shown to derive from peripheral conversion from the androgens rather than to ''accumulation'' resulting from defective removal of these steroids by the diseased liver. Moreover, subacute administration of alcohol to normal volunteers resulted in a fall in the plasma level and production rate of testosterone. Thus, it appears that alcohol per se has significant effects on the metabolism of the sex hormones. Further studies will be presented and the implications of these observations discussed. (Author)

141. Southren, A. L., Gordon, G. G., Olivo, J., Rafii, F., & Rosenthal, W. S. Androgen metabolism in cirrhosis of the liver. *Metabolism,* 1973, *22,* 695–702.

Androgen metabolism was studied in male patients with cirrhosis of the liver. The plasma level, metabolic clearance, and production rates of testosterone were decreased while the conversion ratio and rate transport constant of testosterone to androstenedione were increased. Administration of testosterone produced a marked increase in the metabolic clearance rate of testosterone indicating that parenchymal hepatic dysfunction per se was not the cause for the reduced clearance rate. Moreover, the patients were found to have normal testicular reserve for the biosynthesis of testosterone as indicated by an almost fourfold increase in the plasma concentration of testosterone following the administration of human chorionic gonadotropin. These data demonstrate that the reduced production rate of testosterone in male cirrhotics is not due primarily to testicular disease but possibly reflects hypothalamic-pituitary suppression secondary to increased circulating estrogens. The increase in the rate of conversion of testosterone to androstenedione, found in the present study, is consistent with this hypothesis. The present investigation thus provides quantitative data on the hypogonadal state in cirrhosis and suggests possible mechanisms for the alteration in androgen metabolism. (Author)

142. Van Thiel, D. H. Liver disease and sexual functioning. *Medical Aspects of Human Sexuality,* 1976, *10,* 117–118.

In this article written for physicians who are called upon to advise patients with liver disease and concomitant decrement in sexual functioning, 4 common liver diseases are briefly discussed: infectious hepatitis, serum hepatitis, chronic active hepatitis, and alcoholic liver disease. The author advises physicians to reassure patients that reduced sexual interest is common and temporary with hepatitis. With alcoholic liver disease, sexual functioning may be temporarily disturbed and will not be permanently impaired in males unless there has been irreversible injury to the testes. The author comments that little is known about the effects on women except for menstrual cycle abnormalities but speculates that ovarian damage, analogous to testicular damage, may occur.

143. Van Thiel, D. H. Feminization of chronic alcoholic men: A formulation. *Yale Journal of Biology and Medicine,* 1979, *52,* 219–225.

Theories on feminization of men alcoholics with advanced liver disease and on the pathogenic significance of an altered estrogen : androgen ratio in alcoholic men are reviewed, along with supporting and refuting evidence, and a new hypothesis is deduced. The hypothesis is based on recent findings that the conversion (aromatization) of weak androgens (androstenedione) to estrogens (principally estrone) occurs at many sites and is increased in men with alcoholic cirrhosis; it has been shown that increased peripheral conversion can account for at least 60% of plasma estradiol and estrone in these men. It is hypothesized that in male alcoholics with cirrhosis and portal hypertension with portal-systemic shunting around or through the liver, the steroids cleared from the plasma and reabsorbed in the gut, which are normally rapidly re-excreted into bile, gain access to the systemic circulation. There they maintain estradiol, estrone, and androstenedione levels at normal to moderately increased levels despite advanced gonad failure (common in alcoholic cirrhosis) and reduced production rates. Such reabsorbed steroids can then directly act at peripheral tissues as estrogens or be converted to estrogen. Finally, the net effect of reduced gonadal androgen production and increased estrogen levels due to peripheral conversion may alter tissue sensitivity to estrogens. (RUCAS)

144. Van Thiel, D. H., Gavaler, J. S., Lester, R., Loriaux, D. L., & Braunstein, G. D. Plasma estrone, prolactin, neurophysin, and sex steroid-binding globulin in chronic alcoholic men. *Metabolism,* 1975, *24,* 1015–1019.

Significant elevations of plasma estrone, prolactin, estrogen-stimulated neurophysin, and sex-steroid binding globulin were observed in chronic alcoholic men with varying degrees of alcoholic liver disease. Plasma concentrations of each hormone were elevated at least twofold compared with values obtained for normal men. Concentrations of estrone and prolactin in subjects with gynecomastia were significantly greater than were concentrations of these hormones in those without this physical sign. Similarly, those subjects with spider angiomata had significantly greater plasma estrone levels than did men without this cutaneous vascular abnormality. These findings may provide a partial explanation of the development of feminization in chronic alcoholic men. (NCALI)

145. Van Thiel, D. H., & Lester, R. Sex and alcohol. *New England Journal of Medicine,* 1974, *291,* 251–252.

The development of testicular atrophy, gynecomastia, changes in body hair, and vascular abnormalities observed in male alcoholics with Laennec's cirrhosis has been attributed to sex-steroid imbalance secondary to liver disease. However, feminization has been observed in the absence of liver disease and in patients with normal plasma estrogen levels. The authors offer an alternative hypothesis, a 2-stage development of hypoandrogenicity. Initially, alcohol has direct and indirect reversible effects on testosterone synthesis and spermatogenesis. Ultimately, alcohol ingestion results in irreversible liver and testicular tissue damage which permanently alters metabolism of sex-steroids and produces testicular germ-cell injury.

146. Van Thiel, D. H., & Lester, R. Alcoholism: Its effect on hypothalamic-pituitary-gonadal function. *Gastroenterology,* 1976, *71,* 318–327.

This article reviews research into the effect of alcoholism on hypothalamic-pituitary function. Both as the result of liver disease and of alcoholism per se, chronic alcoholics develop infertility, sterility, gonadal atrophy, hypoandrogenization, and feminization. The hypothalamic-pituitary abnormalities associated with alcoholism include hyperprolactenemia-increased estrogen-stimulated neurophysin levels, suppressed secretion of plasma gonadotropins, and loss of gonadotropin reserve. Several of the possible mechanisms potentially responsible for the development of these endocrine abnormalities are discussed. The rationale for suspecting that alcohol might either interfere with Vitamin A metabolism or alter the redox state of the testes, thus affecting germ cell proliferation and steroidogenesis, is presented. A possible mechanism for sexual changes observed in chronic alcoholic men is proposed. (Author)

147. Van Thiel, D. H., & Lester, R. Sex and alcohol: A second peek. *New England Journal of Medicine,* 1976, *295,* 835–836.

Research on the pathogenesis of feminization of alcoholic men is briefly reviewed, including recent studies confirming the authors' earlier speculation that such feminization might have a dual origin: derivative effects of alcohol-induced liver injury and effects directly related to the ingestion and metabolism of alcohol. It is further speculated that since alcohol dehydrogenase is present in testicular tissue, the demasculinization, diminished plasma testosterone concentration,

and aspermatogenesis commonly associated with the syndrome might be directly attributed to the effects of alcohol on the testes. Two lines of evidence confirming this hypothesis are discussed: (1) studies of alcohol-fed animals and (2) observations of patients ingesting alcohol. New questions in this line of research are raised. (NCALI)

148. Van Thiel, D. H., & Lester, R. The effect of chronic alcohol abuse on sexual function. *Clinics in Endocrinology and Metabolism,* 1979, *8,* 499–510.

Literature on the effect of alcohol and alcoholism on sexual function is reviewed. (RUCAS)

149. Van Thiel, D. H., Lester, R., & Sherins, R. J. Hypogonadism in alcoholic liver disease: Evidence for a double effect. *Gastroenterology,* 1974, *67,* 1188–1199.

Hypothalamic-pituitary-gonadal function was evaluated in 40 males with liver disease to identify an anatomic location and biochemical mechanism responsible for feminization and hypogonadism. Basal plasma concentrations of follicle-stimulating hormone (FSH), luteinizing hormone (LH), estradiol (E), and testosterone (T) were determined. Hormonal responses to clomiphene and chorionic gonadotropin were evaluated. No correlation between degree of liver disease and degree of hormonal derangement was observed. Mean plasma T levels were lower in association with more severe liver damage (p<.05). Both FSH and LH concentrations ranged from normal to moderately elevated and were significantly elevated when compared to normals (p<.01). Plasma E levels were normal or reduced and did not differ significantly from normal. Plasma T was reduced in half of the subjects and differed significantly from normal (p<.01). Responses to clomiphene and exogenous chorionic gonadotropin were markedly diminished in the majority.

150. Van Thiel, D. H., & Loriaux, D. L. Evidence for an adrenal origin of plasma estrogens in alcoholic men. *Metabolism,* 1979, *28,* 536–541.

Plasma concentrations of testosterone, androstenedione, estradiol, estrone, and hydrocortisone were measured in 11 male alcoholics (mean age 45) during sequential and combined gonadal and adrenal suppression and stimulation. (A new agent was added to the previous ones every fourth day.) Six of the alcoholics had cirrhosis, and 8 had testicular atrophy. The men's basal testosterone did not differ from that of 22 age-matched controls. It declined 75% with gonadal suppression (fluoxymesterone, 80 mg/day for 16 days), remained unchanged with added adrenal suppression (dexamethasone, 8 mg/day), and returned to normal with added gonadal stimulation (human chorionic gonadotropin, 5000 U/day) and remained unchanged by added adrenal stimulation (adrenocorticotropic hormone, 80 U/day). Basal estrone in the alcoholics was double the control values (p<.05) and declined 40% in response to gonadal suppression. While estrone did not respond to gonadal stimulation, it rose six-fold in response to adrenal stimulation. Basal androstenedione was normal and responded to manipulation of gonadal and adrenal function. The results indicate that plasma testosterone and estradiol are of gonadal origin, but estrone is partly of gonadal and chiefly of adrenal origin.

They also support the hypothesis that, in alcoholics with liver disease and portosystemic shunts, excessive conversion of androstenedione to estrone occurs at extrahepatic peripheral sites. (RUCAS)

151. Van Thiel, D. H., Sherins, R. J., & Lester, R. *Mechanism of hypogonadism in alcoholic liver disease.* Paper presented at the 24th Annual Meeting of the American Association for the Study of Liver Diseases, Chicago, October 1973.

Thirty-seven men with alcoholic liver disease, ranging from alcoholic hepatitis to end-stage cirrhosis, were studied to define the mechanisms responsible for hypogonadism. Testicular atrophy was present in 19 subjects, gynecomastia was observed in 6, and a female escutcheon was noted in 23 patients. Testicular biopsies from 8 revealed a diffuse reduction of germinal elements in seminiferous tubules and peritubular fibrosis. In contrast, the Leydig cells appeared normal. Results on plasma FSH, plasma testosterone, plasma levels for estradiol, and hypothalamic-pituitary reserves are reported. It is concluded that: (1) feminization and testicular atrophy observed in alcoholic liver disease cannot be explained by excess estradiol per se, and (2) hypogonadism seen in alcoholic liver disease is in part or whole the result of deficient hypothalamic-pituitary function. (NCALI)

II. Nature and Treatment of Sexual Problems among Alcoholics

Introduction
A. Sexual Adjustment Problems of Alcoholics
    1. Both Sexes (or Gender Unspecified)
    2. Females
    3. Males
B. Sex Therapy and Sex Education with Male and Female Alcoholics

Introduction

This chapter addresses the sexual problems commonly associated with chronic, excessive alcohol use. It is divided into 2 sections. The first concentrates on characteristics of sexual adjustment in the alcohol population, and the second focuses on sex education and sex therapy with alcoholics. Publications containing both kinds of information were categorized on the basis of their dominant theme. As a result, many of the entries in the sex education and therapy section contain some information on sexual adjustment as well.

In Section A the reader will find materials on a variety of sexual adjustment issues reported by alcoholics: sexual dysfunction, spouse's withdrawal of sex, and promiscuity and adultery. Entries include reports of empirical research and survey data as well as review and commentary papers. The section begins with the group of publications dealing with the sexual adjustment of alcoholics of both sexes. Some of these provide data collected from male and female alcoholics on sexual adjustment problems, while others are commentary reflecting on alcoholics in general.

The second part of Section A contains information on female alcoholics' sexual behavior patterns. Some of these titles examine the differences observed in alcoholic women's sexual behavior as a function of demographic variables and personality characteristics. Information on sexual dysfunction problems is found here as well. The last part of this section compiles publications on male alcoholics and their sexual adjustment problems. Entries include documentation of the incidence of sexual dysfunction among male alcoholics, observations on the changes in sexual adjustment during sobriety, and research efforts to differentiate organically caused impotence from psychogenic impotence. In addition, articles directed toward physicians and other professionals working with alcoholics alert the professional to signs of marital and sexual difficulties in their patients.

Section B contains a variety of material on sex education and therapy. Some articles address criteria for deciding on the appropriateness of sex therapy, penile prosthesis, or hormone therapy. Others describe the qualities of effective sex education and therapy programs, such as the need for adequate training and self-awareness in staff members. Still others educate the reader on sexual functioning and sex therapy techniques. Case histories and therapy program evaluations also are included in this section.

A. Sexual Adjustment Problems of Alcoholics

1. Both Sexes (or Gender Unspecified)

152. Ablon, J., & Cunningham, W. Implications of cultural patterning for the delivery of alcoholism services. *Journal of Studies on Alcohol*, 1981, (Supplement 9), 185–206.

The significance of culturally patterned family life, attitudes toward sexuality, and parenting behavior in "alcoholic families" has rarely been acknowledged by researchers or by clinicians. This paper describes a specific population of families at high risk for alcohol problems and presents specific directives for the planning and delivery of services. The findings suggest that to understand the role of alcohol use in this population and to plan and implement effective clinical services to meet critical needs, historical and cultural features must be taken into account. Detailed knowledge of family lifestyle is characteristically not gathered by care providers within the traditional clinical context. Thus a model for a multidisciplinary team constituted by an anthropologist-researcher and a clinician is suggested in such very complex and problematic areas of health concern as alcohol misuse. In this manner, sociocultural information may contribute significantly to more effective efforts in the planning and delivery of services. (Author)

153. Al-Anon Family Group Headquarters, Inc. *The dilemma of the alcoholic marriage*. New York: Author, 1971.

This book is written for the nonalcoholic partner, most typically the wife, in an alcoholic marriage. Marital and sexual difficulties commonly observed in alcoholic marriage are discussed in nontechnical language using a straightforward and understanding manner. Sexual dysfunction as a result of active drinking is noted to be common, with secondary impotence developing during periods of sobriety as a result of the alcoholic's perceptions of his sexual failures during periods of active drinking. The process is illustrated with examples of couples having alcohol-related marital and sexual difficulties. Coping strategies for the nonalcoholic partner are discussed.

154. Beckman, L. J. Reported effects of alcohol on the sexual feelings and behavior of women alcoholics and nonalcoholics. *Journal of Studies on Alcohol*, 1979, *40*, 272–282.

The effects of alcohol on sexual feelings and experience, along with reproductive dysfunction, were investigated in 477 persons: 120 female alcoholics; 119 matched female nonalcoholics (normal controls); 118 female nonalcoholics in treatment for psychiatric problems (treatment controls); and 120 male alcoholics. The alcoholics and treatment controls were recruited from treatment facilities in southern California. The alcoholics differed from all others in that the alcoholics, both men and women, were more likely to report enjoying and engaging in sexual intercourse while drinking. All groups reported less inhibition after drinking. More alcoholics than normal controls reported that after drinking they would be more likely to have sexual intercourse with persons with whom they normally would not. More women alcoholics than normal controls reported engaging in sexual acts while drinking that they would not otherwise engage in. Normal controls reported the most sexual satisfaction, while women alcoholics reported the least. Women alcoholics were more likely than normal controls to report having a sexual encounter with someone of the same sex. Reproduction dysfunction was more typical of women having various types of psychopathology, including alcoholism, than of normal women.

155. Benedetti, G. Impotenz und frigidität. [Impotence and frigidity.] *Hexagon Roche*, 1978, *6*, 7–12.

In a survey of psychological causes of impotence and frigidity it is pointed out that alcoholics often have feelings of sexual inferiority, but it is debatable whether this anxiety is responsible for alcoholism or whether, conversely, impotence caused by chronic intoxication triggers the anxiety. There is no doubt, however, that such anxiety can develop into the jealousy mania seen in impotent alcoholics. (RUCAS)

156. Blane, H. T. Sexual problems of alcoholics. *Medical Aspects of Human Sexuality*, 1976, *10*, 103.

The author responds to a reader question about sexual problems of alcoholics in the question and answer section of this journal. He indicates that research findings over the past decade suggest that a diffuse unstable same-sex identity, rather than a cross-sex identification, characterizes alcoholics of both sexes. Men drink to feel more manly and women to feel more feminine. Alcoholics may have specific sexual problems which play a prominent part in the development and maintenance of the drinking problems. These may include covert or overt homosexuality, but just as often they include heterosexual or other sexual difficulties. Sexual problems proceed from the alcoholic condition: reduced sexual drive, alcohol-induced impotence, promiscuity, and brutish sexual relations. Clinical sensitivity to these problems is important in treating alcoholics.

157. Estes, N. J., Smith-DiJulio, K., & Heinemann, M. E. Features of alcoholism: Physiologic and psychosocial aspects. In N. J. Estes, K. Smith-DiJulio, & M. E. Heinemann, *Nursing diagnosis of the alcoholic person.* St. Louis, MO: C. V. Mosby, 1980.

Alcoholic persons differ in the responses they exhibit to excessive alcohol consumption and to the consequences they experience as a result of long-term consumption. Alcohol-associated physiologic and psychosocial deviations for which the alcoholic person is at risk are described in this chapter. The development of hypogonadism, endocrine disturbances, impotence, and other sex-related problems in males is discussed in a section on the genitourinary system. The authors remark that the effects of alcohol on the sexual functioning of women is not known. (Author)

158. Ewing, J. A. Alcohol, sex, and marriage. *Medical Aspects of Human Sexuality,* 1968, *2,* 43–45; 48–50.

This article was written for physicians who encounter alcoholics among the patients they see in their practice. Described are the effects of alcohol on sexual performance, commonly observed marital and family problems (e.g., emotional and sexual conflicts between spouses, implicit or overt incestuous behavior), diagnostic indicators and causes of alcoholism, personality characteristics of the alcoholic, common problems among wives of alcoholics, the alcoholic wife, and the physician's role in treatment. Sexual performance is initially enhanced by alcohol's depressant effect on the rostral parts of the cerebrum which mediate self-control. Excessive amounts of alcohol, however, interfere with performance, which leads to difficulties achieving tumescence and achieving orgasm. Alcohol intoxication may mask existing sexual problems or may complicate them. Treatment of the underlying alcoholism may include disulfiram (Antabuse) treatment, Alcoholics Anonymous, or a weekly, one-hour group meeting with 5–6 alcoholic patients. When the alcoholic patient refuses treatment, unilateral treatment of the nonalcoholic spouse may be called for.

159. Freedberg, E. J., & Scherer, S. E. The Ontario Problem Assessment Battery for alcoholics. *Psychological Reports,* 1977, *40,* 743–746.

Normative data for the Ontario Problem Assessment Battery for alcoholics are reported. Scales on sexual adjustment are included for single alcoholics and for married alcoholics and their spouses. Results indicate that the Battery's content and scaling do not show ceiling effects for either 172 alcoholics or 68 of the spouses. (Ns vary over measures.) Both groups report moderate severity of problems in social coping skills and general lifestyle-related areas. (Author)

160. Gabris, G. Médicaments psychotropes et sexualité. [Psychotropic drugs and sexuality.] *Praxis,* 1979, *68,* 1477–1481.

Alcohol depresses sexual activity although it can cause a feeling of well-being by lifting inhibition. Chronic alcoholism in the long run leads invariably to the abolition of sexual functioning. (RUCAS)

161. Ghodse, A. H., & Tregenza, G. S. The physical effects and metabolism of alcohol. In Camberwell Council on Alcoholism, *Women and alcohol.* New York: Tavistock Publications, 1980.

It seems likely that alcohol may have very different effects on the sexual functions of men and women, although most research on the effect of alcohol on the endocrine system and sexual behavior involves only males. Some effects of chronic, heavy consumption of alcohol on men are discussed (e.g., atrophy of the testicles, impaired sex drive, and fertility). The author then points out that, with the increasing number of alcohol-related problems in women, it is becoming more important to know accurately any specific areas of susceptibility. For example, it has been observed that alcoholic women tend to have a greater number of miscarriages than nonalcoholics. This could be due to a higher conception rate, which in turn could be attributed to a lack of contraceptive measures or to greater sexual activity.

162. Godlewski, J. Problematyka alkoholowa w seksuologii. [Alcoholic problems in sexology.] *Problemy Alkoholizmu,* 1980, *27,* 7–8.

The effects of alcohol abuse on sexual relations (sex drive and performance) and the biological and psychological mechanisms of alcohol action on sexuality are discussed. The widespread belief that alcohol drinking is beneficial to sexual life is disputed. (NCALI)

163. Gomberg, E. S. Drinking patterns of women alcoholics. In V. Burtle (Ed.), *Women who drink: Alcoholic experience and psychotherapy.* Springfield, IL: Charles C. Thomas, 1979.

Findings from various studies are presented regarding: (1) the effects of alcohol on women and on men, (2) male and female alcoholism—manifestations, consequences, and intrasex differences among women, and (3) use of substances other than alcohol by women, used alone or in combination with alcohol. Alcohol effects on blood alcohol levels, on sexuality, and on reproductive systems are considered. Seven methods for classifying women with alcohol problems are presented for studying intrasex differences. Findings are reviewed with the warning that generalizations are suspect because they can only apply to certain subgroups of alcoholics. (NCALI)

164. Hollister, L. E. Drugs and sexual behavior in man. *Life Sciences,* 1975, *17,* 661–668.

Drugs for treating diminished sexual function remain largely unsatisfactory, but new basic knowledge about the roles of the neurotransmitters, dopamine and serotonin, may allow the formulation of more effective compounds. Drugs for decreasing sexual activity are more numerous and more effective although far less desired. The antiandrogen, cyproterone, is being studied as a treatment for sexual offenders. Drugs used for treatment of nonsexual disorders may have sexual effects, and information should be collected about concurrent drug-taking in anyone with a complaint about sexual function. Sympatholytics, ganglionic blocking drugs, antipsychotics, and lithium may all impair sexual functions. Of the social drugs, alcohol is most clearly deleterious in its effects; the sexual consequences of prolonged alcohol abuse in men and women are noted briefly. Much mystique has grown about the use of illicit social drugs as sexual stimulants. Except for their effects as disinhibiting agents, little rationale exists for most of the claims made. Like alcohol, heroin and other opiates decrease sexual activity. Amphetamines are best documented as sexual stimulants, although such effects usually require substantial doses. (Author)

165. Katz, A., Morgan, M. Y., & Sherlock, S. Alcoholism treatment in a medical setting. *Journal of Studies on Alcohol*, 1981, *42*, 136–143.

Twenty-one men and 15 women hospitalized in the medical unit of the Royal Free Hospital, London, for alcohol-related liver disease were monitored by a physician and a clinical psychologist for 6 months after discharge. The patients had a mean age of 45; 29 were British in origin, 14 were married, 11 were professionals or managers, and 16 had a family history of alcoholism. Each patient was urged to make an outpatient visit to the psychologist once a week and to visit the medical outpatient department when necessary. All were asked to keep a record of each drink consumed. Mean daily consumption, calculated at each outpatient visit, was verified by contacting the patients' relatives and close friends. Random measurements of blood alcohol concentration were made. Patients were offered marital, vocational, and other counseling, when appropriate, and were urged to curb their drinking. At the end of 6 months, 17 of the 36 were abstaining, 8 had reduced their daily intake to less than 50 g of absolute alcohol, and 11 were still misusing alcohol. Continued misuse of alcohol was significantly related (p=.04) to the presence of an alcoholic partner and to sexual dysfunction (p<.05). (RUCAS)

166. Krimmel, H. E. The alcoholic and his family. In P.G. Bourne & R. Fox (Eds.), *Alcoholism: Progress in research and treatment*. New York: Academic Press, 1973.

This chapter describes the disrupted family functioning of the alcoholic and the anguish experienced by all family members, including the alcoholic. In sexual relationships, alcoholism creates problems that have repercussions in the total life of the family. The female alcoholic, unlike the male, is able to perform sexually and she may barter sex for alcohol. The male alcoholic is often impotent while drinking. His wife may feel repulsed by him in his drunken state and be unable to respond to him sexually. Repeated incidents of impotence, repulsion, or both are cumulative and carry over into periods of sobriety. The author sees the alcoholic husband as drifting into dependency, which in turn emphasizes inadequacies. In an effort to assert himself and reestablish his dominance he may become belligerent, abusive, and demanding. In addition, the author points out that wives may withhold sex until the drinking stops in order to control the alcoholic husbands' drinking behavior.

167. Krzyzowski, J., & Thille, Z. Zaburzenia zycia plciowego w alkoholizmie. [Sex-life disorders in alcoholism.] In T. Bilikiewicz (Ed.), *Problemy seksuologii*. Warsaw: Panotwowy Zaklad Wydawnictw Llkarskich, 1965.

168. Levine, J. The sexual adjustment of alcoholics: A clinical study of a selected sample. *Quarterly Journal of Studies on Alcohol*, 1955, *16*, 675–680.

The clinical records of 79 patients at an alcoholism outpatient clinic, chosen from 400 cases for completeness of their files, were examined. The sample consisted of 63 males and 16 females. A majority showed diminished interest in heterosexual relationships. Of the males: 12 denied all sexual activity, 44 had sexual intercourse once every 3 months or less, 2 were homosexuals, 19 stated sexual activity was as frequent as once or twice a week, and all but 5 of these had some sexual problem. Of the women studied: 8 had no heterosexual relations, 3 claimed frequent intercourse but were reported by their therapist to be frigid, 5 were promiscuous, and each reported almost complete absence of orgasm. The effects of alcohol on sex drive are not uniform. In most there is a diminution of drive, but some become increasingly demanding. Where drive increases, there are suggestions of impaired performance. Nearly 75% of the men had had a strongly dominant, overprotective mother and a relatively weak, distant, or absent father toward whom hostility was felt. In many instances a dependence on the mother was clear. Strong feminine identification and attraction for members of the same sex is understandable. Homosexuality is occasionally overt under the influence of alcohol but in most cases is so taboo as to be completely repressed. (RUCAS)

169. McFalls, J. A., Jr. Alcoholism. In J. A. McFalls, Jr. (Ed.), *Psychopathology and Subfecundity*. New York: Academic Press, 1979.

In this literature review, alcoholism is defined as a personality disorder, first, and a drug abuse disorder, second. From this point of view, the author describes the relationships between alcoholism and subfecundity: reverse causal—sexual dysfunction and infertility precipitate chronic, excessive use of alcohol; direct causal—interference of alcohol with hormone metabolism and/or spermatogenesis; intervening causal—alcoholism causes medical disorders that in turn lead to sexual dysfunction and reduced fertility; spurious causal—psychopathology may be the primary cause of subfecundity; and alcoholism may be a correlate of the psychopathology. The mechanisms by which alcoholism is seen to cause subfecundity are coital inability, conceptive failure, and pregnancy loss. Alcoholism affects fecundity indirectly through its detrimental effect on coital frequency and the marital relationship. Also, alcoholic women are counseled to avoid childbearing due to the risk of fetal alcohol syndrome.

170. Molcan, J., Strecko, A., Nábelek, L'., & Hlava, K. Prieskum sexuálnej aktivity alkoholikov a alkoholiciek. [Research of the sexual activity of male and female alcoholics.] *Protialkoholický Obzor,* 1978, *13,* 1–13.

Fifty-four chronic alcoholics were examined and observed. The average age of the patients was 38. The drinking period of males was 15 years, that of women 11 years. There were 45% married men, 58% married women, 24% unmarried men, 17% unmarried women, 31% divorced men, 25% divorced women; 64% of the men and 92% of the women had permanent partners; 59% of the men and 92% of the women had conflicts in the partnership; and 92% of the men and all the women stated the abuse of alcohol as the main reason for the disintegration of their marriages. The results were compared with the results from 35 psychically healthy persons. All the observed persons were examined psychiatrically, and sexual function was specially quantified by means of Mellan's questionnaire, which enabled the evaluations of apotency and sexual activity, the process of coitus, an emotional aspect and self-evaluation, and the duration of sexual defect. According to the results, defects of sexual function were shown in all of its components in chronic intoxication of men. While there was relatively little effect on the need and frequency of sexual relaxation and sexual function, there was a relatively greater effect on the orgasmic ability and the mood after coitus. On the basis of this, the development of anesthetic-frigid syndrome in the process of intoxication may be confirmed. In the control group of women, less sexual activity than in the case of men was observed on the border of the norm. (English abstract and English title were provided as a summary at the end of foreign article cited above.) (Author)

171. Pashchenkov, S. Z. O klinicheskom techenii alkogolizma u bolnykh s semeinoi otyagoshchennostyu. [The clinical evolution of alcoholism in patients with a familial taint.] *Klinicheskaia Meditsina,* 1974, *52,* 93–96.

Of a group of 3,332 alcoholics hospitalized during 1967–72, of whom 1,027 had one alcoholic parent, 84 patients (68 women) were selected for an investigation of the clinical course of familial alcoholism. These patients came from homes in which they were exposed from early childhood to the continuous example and encouragement of excessively drinking parents and close relatives; 61 of the 68 women were married to alcoholics. About 38% of the 84 patients started drinking between ages 14 and 18; 42% between 19 and 20; and 19% between 21 and 25. The first withdrawal syndrome occurred in 31 patients during the first year of excessive drinking, in 42 during the second year, and in only 11 during the third year. The clinical course was characterized by a very rapid progression from the neurasthenic stage of alcoholism to the addictive and finally encephalopathic stage (the 3 stages of alcoholism in the Soviet classification); 63.4% had severe forms of alcoholism at ages 20–30. Profound changes in character, personality, and behavior occurred within 2 to 3 years of heavy drinking, producing a rapid disintegration of occupational, social, and marital life. The women suffered from menstrual disturbances, inflammation of the adnexa uteri, ectopic pregnancies, frigidity, and sterility; the men from libido reduction and impotence; both men and women suffered from considerable damage to the cardiovascular system and gastrointestinal tract. (RUCAS)

172. Pollmer, E. *Alcoholic personalities.* New York: Exposition Press, 1965.

During the years of World War II, the author undertook a study of alcoholics in Paris' skid row district. Information on intelligence, school and occupational performance, family background, and sexuality was collected from approximately 840 male and 600 female alcoholics. This book contains extensive descriptive information on the sexual adjustment of male and female alcoholics. Subjects were classified into 6 categories: males of superior, average, and inferior intelligence, and females of superior, average, and inferior intelligence. Subjects within each category showed consistencies in drinking habits, education, family background, sex education, and sexual behavior which differentiated each category from the others. Homosexuality, prostitution, promiscuity, or sexual deviance was more characteristic of some groups than others. Nonalcoholic neurotics with characteristics similar to the alcoholics were also studied for comparison, and attempts were made to induce alcoholism among them. The neurotics did not become alcoholics. Major differences between the neurotics and the alcoholics were that the neurotics were able to pinpoint problems and take aggressive action. The alcoholics on the other hand experienced free-floating anxiety, which they sought to drown with alcohol. Sexuality was often an important factor in the alcoholics' anxiety in all classifications. Sexuality was a particularly important causative factor for the alcoholism among subjects of superior intelligence. For the males in this group, sexual reeducation played an important role in their recovery from alcoholism.

173. Powell, D. J. Sexual dysfunction and alcoholism. *Journal of Sex Education and Therapy,* 1980, *6,* 40–46.

Literature on the relationship between sexual dysfunction and alcohol abuse is reviewed (80 items); particular attention is paid to psychological and physiological variables that may contribute to sexual dysfunction. The alcoholic marriage, the effects of alcohol abuse on the sexuality of the man and woman, as well as the implications of these findings for treatment and training, are examined. It is suggested that alcoholism and sex counselors cannot function autonomously, each neglecting the sphere of the other. (RUCAS)

174. Rathod, N. H., & Thomson, I. G. Women alcoholics: A clinical study. *Quarterly Journal of Studies on Alcohol,* 1971, *32,* 45–52.

Social and personal histories and characteristics were compared in 30 female and 30 male alcoholics, patients at the Graylingwell Hospital, Chichester, England, matched in age (45 and 47 years) and social class. Eighteen of the women and 12 of the men had alcoholic parents (p<.05); 13 and 2 respectively had lost a parent before age 16 (p<.001); 8 and 2 had experienced a broken engagement (p<.05); 19 and 15 had had a broken marriage; 6 and 2 had illegitimate children; 11 and 2 had attempted suicide (p<.01); 10 and 0 had been treated for mental illness before the onset of problem drinking (p<.001); 9 and 6 had married problem drinkers; and 7 and 10 had been convicted of a crime (the female:male ratio in the U. K. is 1:12). In addition, repeated infidelity was found to have occurred in 10 of the women and 15 of the men; the difference is not significant. However, when viewed in conjunction with alcoholism, 5 of the women and 2 of the men reported repeated infidelity before the onset of problem drinking, and in 5 women and 13 men it had occurred only after the onset of problem drinking. Thus, men alcoholics seem to be more repeatedly unfaithful than do women alcoholics (p<.05). A corollary of this is the suggestion that women destined to become alcoholics are more frequently unfaithful in marriage before the onset of problem drinking. The women had evidently suffered more childhood deprivation and were more maladjusted than the men. (Author)

175. Renshaw, D. C. Sexual problems of alcoholics. *Chicago Medicine,* 1975, *78,* 433–436.

The stereotype of the sexually liberal alcoholic is an inaccurate generalization. Moderate drinking facilitates sexual behavior by lowering inhibitions. However, large amounts depress central nervous system synchronization of sexual activity. Excessive alcohol ingestion can produce sexual dysfunction in both sexes. Males may become impotent under the influence of alcohol, which may generate enough anxiety to produce secondary psychogenic impotence persisting in sober periods. Some female alcoholics report inability to achieve orgasm and reduced interest in sex; others report involvement in prostitution, promiscuity, and arrests for sexual misconduct. Among male alcoholics, 40%–60% are said to have potency problems. Alcohol interferes with sexual functioning by its effects on the central nervous system, the autonomic nervous sytem, peripheral nerves, the vascular system and the endocrine system. Physical concomitants of alcohol abuse, i.e., peripheral neuropathy, liver damage, and diabetes mellitus, contribute to organic impotence. However, a definitive diagnosis of organic vs. psychogenic sexual dysfunction is not always possible. The point is illustrated with a case history.

176. Renshaw, D. C. Drugs and sex: A study of the effect of drugs on human sexuality. *Nursing Care,* 1978, *11,* 16–19.

In a description of the effects of various drugs and medicines on sex drive and sexual functioning, it is noted that moderate social drinking facilitates sexual exchange, but that alcohol may also cause an occasional episode of impotence or partial erection. The anxiety thus generated may persist long after the alcohol has been eliminated. (RUCAS)

177. Sclare, A. B. Alcoholism in doctors. *British Journal of Alcohol and Alcoholism,* 1979, *14,* 181–196.

There were 30 alcoholics (mean age 17; 3 women) among 100 psychiatrically ill doctors treated in Glasgow between 1958 and 1977. General practitioners made up 60% of the alcoholics, who also suffered from personality disorders, drug dependence, depression, psychosexual problems, delirium tremens, and anxiety neurosis. Follow-up of the alcoholics 3–16 years later (mean 7.4 years) indicated that 25 were still registered practitioners. (RUCAS)

178. Sexual dysfunction in the alcoholic male. *Alcoholism,* September-October 1980, pp. 28–31.

In an interview, Dr. Richard Morin discusses the insights he gained from personal experience as a recovering alcoholic and as a physician specializing in alcoholism and drug abuse-related problems. Sexual problems begin as drinking becomes heavier. Ignorance of the relationship between sex and alcohol is common. Alcohol's influence on physiological mechanisms involved in sexual responding can have long-term effects. Males become impotent and females become anorgasmic. Efforts to enliven sexuality can lead to adultery or promiscuity. Male alcoholics may experience "homosexual panic"; females may blame their husbands for their unsatisfying sexual experiences. Recovery of sexual function begins soon after achieving sobriety. Factors influencing the rate of recovery are the degree of damage caused by alcohol, performance anxiety, hostility between spouses, and marital problems. Sex therapy may be called for.

179. Smith, J. W. Libido of female alcoholics. *Medical Aspects of Human Sexuality,* 1975, *9,* 99.

The author responds to a reader question about the loss of libido in women who are abstinent 1 to 2 years after 10 to 15 years of heavy drinking. He indicates that complaints of loss of libido are rare among women alcoholics. Since depression is well known to affect libido adversely and is relatively common in women alcoholics, it should be one of the first factors considered in loss of libido. The sexual drive is likewise preserved in men alcoholics; those complaining of impotence have a neurophysiological defect that impedes erection. (RUCAS)

180. Steinglass, P. An experimental treatment program for alcoholic couples. *Journal of Studies on Alcohol,* 1979, *40,* 159–182.

Ten couples in which at least 1 member was an alcoholic were treated in an experimental 6-week program that included a period of conjoint hospitalization. Alcohol was freely available for the first 7 days of the 10-day hospitalization period, and the couples were encouraged to reproduce as closely as possible their usual drinking and interactional behavior. A battery of evaluative instruments (Chronological Drinking Record, SCL-90, Structured and Scaled Interview to Assess Maladjustment, Inventory of Marital Conflict, Subject is Marriage) were administered to the subjects just before therapy and 6 months after therapy to assess changes in both individual and marital behavior. The results failed to demonstrate a consistent pattern of positive behavioral change. All couples reported negative change or no change from pre- to posttherapy on the sexual satisfaction scale of the marriage questionnaire. Nevertheless, several trends did emerge: (a) modest positive changes occurred in drinking patterns of alcoholics; (b) a strong correlation was demonstrated between reduction in drinking by the alcoholic and reduction in psychiatric symptomatology in the nonalcoholic spouse; (c) marked changes in interactional behavior were noted after therapy, but they did not follow consistent directions; (d) the two therapists involved in the program had different degrees of success in producing behavioral changes. It is concluded that the results support the systems model of alcoholism, which proposes that alcoholism is a family-level process, and that the use of alcohol during treatment can be a useful means for the therapist and the patient to gain insight into the drinking problem. (RUCAS)

181. Stump, D. *Alcohol and sex.* Unpublished report prepared by the Colorado Task Force on Alcoholism, 1979. (Available from Rockville, MD: National Clearinghouse for Alcohol Information, Report No. NCAI044079.)

The effects of alcohol on sexual performance, desire, and behavior are discussed. (NCALI)

182. Tamerin, J. S. Alcoholism and family discord. *Medical Aspects of Human Sexuality,* 1979, *13,* 143–144.

The author advises physicians to be prepared to work with the entire family, particularly the spouse, when dealing with alcoholism. Further advice includes suggestions for exploring the effects of alcohol on both spouses' level of sexual interest. The possibility that alcohol is a means of avoiding sex, thereby masking an underlying sexual problem, is also mentioned.

183. Watts, R. J. The physiological interrelationships between depression, drugs, and sexuality. *Nursing Forum,* 1978, *17,* 168–183.

This article reviews evidence indicating an interaction between depression, drugs, and sexual impairment. Alcohol used in excessive amounts selectively depresses various parts of the cerebral cortex, reduces inhibition, and gives the individual greater freedom for sexual expression. However, among males, extensive alcohol abuse eventually causes impotence and ejaculatory dysfunction. Alcohol-induced impotence can initiate a vicious cycle by generating fears of impotence which interfere with sexual performance while sober. Prolonged alcohol abuse leads to anatomical and endocrine disturbances that disrupt erectile function and reduce libido. Many female alcoholics also complain of diminished sexual interest and orgasmic dysfunction. Sexual impairment may also be due to a destructive interpersonal relationship between the alcoholic and spouse.

184. Williams, K. H. An overview of sexual problems in alcoholism. In J. Newman (Ed.), *Sexual counseling for persons with alcohol problems: Proceedings of a workshop at Pittsburgh, Pennsylvania, January 22-23, 1976.* Pittsburgh, PA: University of Pittsburgh, 1976.

Sexual dysfunctioning in the alcoholic (the inability of the alcoholic to have satisfactory interpersonal sexual relationships) is discussed. The physiological effect of alcohol on sexual performance can cause premature ejaculation, frigidity, and various kinds of impotence. These are described along with the sexual problems encountered by the alcoholic homosexual. If therapy is to be successful in such cases, it is suggested that the therapist come to grips with his/her own sexuality to foster an atmosphere of honesty and open discussion with the alcoholic patient.

2. Females

185. Barnes, J. L., Benson, C. S., & Wilsnack, S. C. Psychosocial characteristics of women with alcoholic fathers. In M. Galanter (Ed.), *Currents in Alcoholism* (Vol. 6). New York: Grune & Stratton, 1979.

Psychosocial characteristics of young women at "high risk" were investigated on the basis of their fathers' alcoholism for the development of a number of problems, including alcoholism. Subjects were college women enrolled in undergraduate classes at Indiana University. Five areas of inquiry were selected for study: (1) drinking behavior and attitudes, (2) affective disorder, especially depression, (3) sex role characteristics, (4) sexual behavior and attitudes, and (5) perceptions of self and parents. Results indicated that not only do daughters of alcoholics drink more, they also tend to experience more drinking-related problems, and they are more likely to drink for "personal effects." Results did not support the hypotheses that daughters of alcoholic fathers differ from daughters of nonalcoholic fathers on depression and sex-role orientation, and no clear evidence was found of sexual maladjustment among alcoholics' daughters. Clear evidence was found that daughters of alcoholics perceived their fathers differently from daughters of nonalcoholics. Limitations of this study are briefly discussed. (NCALI)

186. Brown, R. A. Controlled drinking training with a female alcoholic. *British Journal of Social Clinical Psychology,* 1978, *17,* 153–157.

Controlled drinking training based upon an avoidance conditioning paradigm has previously been demonstrated to offer an alternative to abstinence for some alcoholics. This paper describes the treatment and outcome of controlled drinking training as applied to a 33-year-old female who had previously attempted abstinence and who could engage in sexual intercourse only after drinking. The subject received 4 weeks of routine inpatient psychotherapy before volunteering for a 6-week controlled drinking training program. She received a total of 14 training sessions during which time she could order whatever she wanted to drink and the drinks were free. She was required to order single measures of drinks with mixers, take small sips, and consume no more than 2 drinks per hour. For 9 of the sessions, finger electrodes were attached to the thumb and forefinger of her nondominant hand. Drinking behavior was rapidly shaped to acceptable social limits. Concomitant with gaining control over drinking, the subject's behavior changed on the ward, becoming more open and involved. Follow-up over a 2-year period found that the subject was able to engage in sexual behavior without drinking and at the end of 2 years was considering marriage.

187. Corrigan, E. M. Women and problem drinking: Notes on beliefs and facts. In D. Robinson (Ed.), *Alcohol problems: Reviews, research and recommendations.* New York: Macmillan, 1979. (Reprinted from *Addictive Diseases: an International Journal,* 1974, *1,* 215–222.)

A review of the research on alcoholic women is presented. The magnitude of the problem, life situations that trigger the onset of problem drinking in women, sexual adjustment, troubles due to excessive alcohol consumption, and treatment outcomes are discussed. The author concludes that the most important factors in determining basic characteristics of female alcoholism include an understanding of the onset and course of progressive drinking in women, the consequences of drinking for themselves and those closest to them, and treatment outcome. Knowledge of possible difference between female and male alcoholism is felt to be essential so that correspondingly different treatment and prevention methods can be put into effect.

188. Curran, F. J. Personality studies in alcoholic women. *Journal of Nervous and Mental Disease*, 1937, *86*, 645–667.

This work represents a study of the sociological and psychological problems in 50 female alcoholics who were selected for this study either because they had alcoholic psychoses or because they were known chronic alcoholics who had many admissions to the alcoholic ward of the Psychopathic Division of Bellevue Hospital. Sixteen of these patients were nonpsychotic. In studying the hallucinatory content, 31 additional cases were used, providing a study of psychotic material in 65 patients. Five detailed case studies are given. It was found that the content of the hallucinations tends to bring out in detail the personality traits already learned or hinted at from the personality studies. The sexual content of the hallucinations were predominantly in connection with heterosexual accusations in contrast to the homosexual accusations in male alcoholics. The threats by the voices not only dealt with the removal of the receptive sex organs but also with general cutting or hurting of the body (dismembering motive). The findings enumerated indicate that a strong attachment to a parent of the same sex, strong narcissism, and strong inner-tensions that make social contact difficult are the outstanding features in the alcoholic women. Alcoholic women are always striving for social recognition and fear that this will not be given. In their acute psychoses they often experience an attack of criticism from others that is a projection of the self-criticism at the base of their social shyness. The alcoholism also influences the aggressive and sadistic tendencies so that in the acute hallucinosis they believe relatives or others have been killed. The alcoholics experience feelings of sexual inferiority and project it in hallucinations to the outside world. (Author)

189. Densen-Gerber, J. Addiction and female sexuality. *Focus on Women—Journal of Addictions and Health*, 1981, *2*, 94–115.

In this discussion of addiction (including alcoholism) and female sexuality, the following topics are addressed: (1) defining healthy human sexuality, (2) current concepts of sexuality, and (3) therapy of human sexual problems. (NCALI)

190. Deshaies, G. Aspects psychiques de alcoolisme chez la femme. [Psychological aspects of alcoholism in women.] *Vie Medicale*, 1965, *46*, 1739–1747.

A 1962 study in France of hospitalized alcoholic women suggests that rejected femininity leads to sexual maladjustment with sadomasochistic marital relationships. (NCALI)

191. De Vito, R. Sex drive in alcoholic women. *Sexuality and Disability*, 1981, *4*, 258.

In response to a reader's question, "Do alcoholic women lose interest in sex?" the author writes that female alcoholics lose interest in sex as their alcohol abuse progresses. This loss may be linked with the effects of alcohol or its metabolites on parts of the brain.

192. Dowsling, J. L. *Women: Alcoholism and sexuality*. Paper presented at the National Council on Alcoholism Annual Meeting, Seattle, May 1980.

Research findings on the specific causes of drinking problems in women are reviewed. These include sex-role conflict, feelings of personal inadequacy, the onset of depression or other emotional problems, specific life crises, and marital disruption. Sexual dysfunction is linked to alcoholism in women on the basis that low self-esteem is a key factor in both alcohol dependency and sexual dysfunction. Characteristics of 3 types of sexual dysfunction are outlined, and the relationship of alcohol to such problems is described. Since sexual dysfunctions are commonly expressed by the recovering alcoholic woman and may have a direct bearing on her potential for recovery, sex therapy is recommended as a direct behavioral therapy that attempts to deal comprehensively with environmental, interpersonal, and organic factors. Sex therapy techniques are discussed. (NCALI)

193. Evans, S., & Schaefer, S. *Why women's sexuality is important to address in chemical dependency treatment programs*. Paper presented at the National Council on Alcoholism Annual Meeting, Seattle, May 1980.

Empirical evidence is reviewed which documents the significant relationship between drug addiction or alcoholism and areas of female sexuality such as incest, sexual assault, sexual preference, and sexual dysfunction. The physiological, psychological, social, and spiritual factors that enter into this relationship are discussed in detail. Efforts made to address sexual concerns at the Chrysalis chemical dependency treatment program in Minneapolis, Minnesota, are described. (NCALI)

194. Gomberg, E. S. Women and alcoholism. In V. Franks & V. Burtle (Eds.), *Women in therapy*. New York: Brunner/Mazel, 1974.

This chapter reviews the literature concerning many facets of alcoholism in women. The section on sexual adjustment contrasts the notion that women with drinking problems are promiscuous with the suggestion that lack of sexual interest is probably more common. The latter is supported by the observation that female alcoholics tend to drink at home, alone or with husbands. Promiscuity may be related to social class, locale of drinking, and drinking partners and not necessarily an inevitable concomitant of alcoholism. For instance, common law marriage and prostitution occur more frequently in a prison population than they do in an outpatient population.

195. Gomberg, E. S. Problems with alcohol and other drugs. In E. S. Gomberg (Ed.), *Gender and disordered behavior; sex differences in psychopathology* (Vol. 15). New York: Brunner/Mazel, 1979.

This review (about 150 bibliographic items) examines: gender differences in substance use in general, and alcohol use in particular; drunkenness as a social phenomenon; the epidemiology and etiology of problem drinking; the antecedents of alcoholism (biological, social, and behavioral); alcoholic behavior; consequences of alcoholism; and treatment and rehabilitation of women. Women use alcohol less often than men to alleviate anxiety; but when they drink, they more often cite "health" reasons. They are also more concerned with alcohol-related health problems. Although more women drink now, it is unclear how this relates to statistics on problem drinking and alcoholism. So far, the male-female ratio among alcoholics still seems to be 4 or 5 to 1. However, among those under 20 admitted to New York state hospitals with a primary diagnosis of alcoholism, the proportion of women is higher than in any other age group. Both women and men show the highest proportion of heavy drinkers in the 45–49 age group, but women have another peak at ages 21–24, which is attributed to dating and mate-seeking behaviors. After the same amount of alcohol, young women reach higher blood alcohol levels than young men. These levels seem to vary with the menstrual cycle and are higher in the premenstrual period. High risk factors for alcoholism in women include childhood deprivation and disruption of early family relationships, heavy or escape drinking and peer pressure to drink, traumatic life events or crises, social environment stresses (within the family or from a woman's role and status in the community), and low self-esteem. Women alcoholics may be divided into early- (teens or 20s) and late-onset (30s–40s) types. Women are much less often arrested for drunkenness than men (1:14), more often divorced or separated when seen for alcoholism treatment; and more frequently drink alone. They come to treatment for different reasons than men. (RUCAS)

196. Hayek, M. A. *Recovered alcoholic women with and without incest experience: A comparative study.* Unpublished doctoral dissertation, Reed University, 1980.

Thirty recovered female alcoholics (aged 17–62) who were at least one year alcohol-free and who had experienced incest were compared with 30 recovered alcoholics without incest experience. No between-group difference was found in family background and psychological functioning. The women of the incest group were significantly more likely to have a mother who is unresponsive to the father ($p<.04$) and to come from a family in which there is parental conflict ($p<.07$). These women were less likely to respect their father ($p<.009$) but were prone to be physically attracted to him ($p<.03$); they were also prone to experience dyspareunia ($p<.03$) and vaginismus ($p<.05$) with sexual intercourse ($p<.05$). They were likely to have felt guilt from the past at the onset of drinking ($p<.001$), to drink at a very young age ($p<.01$), and to feel uncomfortable during sexual encounters if alcohol were not available ($p<.01$). (RUCAS)

197. Homiller, J. D. Alcoholism among women. *Chemical Dependencies: Behavioral and Biomedical Issues,* 1980, *4,* 1–31.

Poor design, inadequate or biased sampling procedures, lack of control groups, contradictory conclusions, and failure to differentiate distinct subgroups of women mark the research literature on alcoholism in women. In addition, there are few attempts to translate the implications of reported differences between men and women into appropriate treatment approaches. Women's self-perceptions must be considered more carefully, especially in designing treatment, and theories on the etiology of women's alcoholism must be tested. Researchers have not properly separated the effects of excessive use of alcohol on women's sexuality and functioning from difficulties in such functioning that may cause, precede, or be independent of alcohol misuse. Treatment outcome measures and criteria are often inappropriate for women who are full-time wives, mothers, or students. Future research must devise methodologies for discerning critical variables of the character of female alcoholism. Attempts must be made to match men and women on socioeconomic status and other critical variables such as age and education. The absence of specific information is a barrier to developing the required public policy. (RUCAS)

198. Johnson, S., & Garzon, S. R. Alcoholism and women. *American Journal of Drug and Alcohol Abuse,* 1978, *5,* 107–122.

The research literature on alcoholism in women is reviewed. The authors note that the unconstrained sexual activity of alcoholic women may be a myth as the research shows that many female alcoholics report a lack of interest in sex. Research is called for to study the effects of alcohol on women's sexuality, particularly in the area of sex hormone metabolism in relationship to ethanol metabolism.

199. Kinsey, B. A. Psychological factors in alcoholic women from a state hospital sample. *American Journal of Psychiatry,* 1968, *124,* 1463–1466.

A state hospital sample of 46 female alcoholics is compared to alcoholic women from higher socioeconomic groups. The data support the contention that a basic psychopathology underlies female alcoholism despite widespread social and cultural differences. This includes childhood experiences with cold, rejecting, domineering mothers and indulgent, ineffective fathers, resulting in a deep sense of personal inadequacy and a lack of preparation for adult roles. Sexual instruction was inadequate. Frigidity, sexual conflicts, and other psychosexual disturbances dominated female alcoholics' relationships. Alcohol is valued for its ability to enable the respondent to be the type of person she "wants to be." There is some support for the view that the crucial factor in female alcoholism is the woman's identification with her father and the concomitant tendency to accept his pattern of drinking. (Author)

200. Kuttner, R. E., & Lorincz, A. B. Promiscuity and prostitution in urbanized Indian communities. *Mental Hygiene*, 1970, *54*, 79–91.

Data on about 100 prostitutes, most of whom were Indians, in the skid row area of Omaha, NE, were obtained from informants and observation. Alcoholism was the primary reason for passing from promiscuity to prostitution. The need for a drink brings these women out early in the day looking for a "mark." By late morning they usually have adequate funds for drinking and socializing in the bars for the rest of the day. Weekends are often spent drinking with relatives or old friends and at all-night drinking parties. Although many of the women have short periods of extra-legal marriage or useful employment, during which they abstain from alcohol, they eventually relapse into prostitution because the entire social life of the skid row area revolves around the taverns. Once drinking begins again, prostitution follows. Rehabilitation would require the early retirement of prostitutes to a stable relationship, with substitute economic opportunities. Recognition of the role of alcoholism is a prerequisite. Prevention of the problem requires early intervention to counteract the debasing influences found in a poverty-ridden ghetto. (RUCAS)

201. Lisansky, E. S. Alcoholism in women: Social and psychological concomitants. *Quarterly Journal of Studies on Alcohol*, 1957, *18*, 588–623.

A comparative study was made of 46 female versus 55 male alcoholics who had at least 2 contacts with outpatient clinics of the Connecticut Commission on Alcoholism. Some of the viewpoints about the alcoholic woman which had been held by earlier investigators were corroborated by the present study. First, it appears that among female alcoholics excessive drinking is precipitated by a definite traumatic event more often than among males. Second, some evidence was found to support the hypothesis that women begin to drink later in life and that when they do become alcoholics, the shift from controlled to uncontrolled drinking is more rapid than for the male alcoholic. Third, on the point that alcoholism in women and sexual promiscuity are somehow related, the data of the present study suggest that sexual promiscuity is associated more frequently with one particular group of female alcoholics than with another. The stereotype of the promiscuous female alcoholic may be based to a large extent on observations of women who display their alcoholism publicly and who get into difficulty with the law. Fourth, on the postulated relationship between feminine physiological function and alcoholism, the age range and time patterns of drinking of the female alcoholics in the present study indicate that there is no simple relationship between excessive drinking, premenstrual tensions, and menopausal difficulties.

202. Lisansky, E. S. The woman alcoholic. *Annals of the American Academy of Political and Social Sciences*, 1958, *315*, 73–81.

Evidence of increased alcoholism among women is discussed, and various ideas about alcoholic women are summarized. In a section on sexual promiscuity, the stereotypic association between promiscuity and alcoholism is discussed in the light of data suggesting that alcoholic women tend to be sexually inhibited and that promiscuity may be associated with a particular subgroup of alcoholic women. The author describes her findings from a study in which she compared: (a) 37 alcoholic women incarcerated in Connecticut penal institutions and 46 alcoholic women who were voluntary outpatients at alcoholism clinics in Connecticut; and (b) 55 male alcoholics who were voluntary outpatients at alcoholism clinics in Connecticut. Variables examined are: social background, early homelife, present family structure, history and patterns of drinking. The 2 groups of alcoholic women differed significantly on many aspects of the variables explored. One difference was that the prison women were more likely to report promiscuity as a concomitant of their drinking. The female and male alcoholics had many significant differences also. No data on sex are reported for the comparisons between male and female alcoholics.

203. Lolli, G. Alcoholism in women. *Connecticut Review on Alcoholism*, 1953, *5*, 9–11.

The author compares the differences between male and female alcoholics, stating: (a) women are more tied to their biology, with their menstrual cycles and menopause creating distress that is remedied with excessive drinking, and (b) women experience a higher incidence of venereal disease due to the fact that alcohol intoxication makes them more vulnerable to sexual attack. Sexual maladjustment frequently accompanies alcohol addiction. Alcohol-related experiences become more important then sexual experiences. Minor sexual difficulties may be magnified in the mind of the alcoholic woman. Some alcoholic women may appear well adjusted while sober but become antagonistic toward the opposite sex while intoxicated. Others who are sexually inhibited while sober may experience a weakening of inhibitions under the influence of alcohol.

204. Mantek, M. Alkoholismus bei frauen. [Alcoholism in women.] *Psychologie Heute*, October 1977, pp. 39–46. (English translation available from Selected Translations of International Alcoholism Research (STIAR), National Clearinghouse for Alcohol Information, P.O. Box 2345, Rockville, MD 20852.)

Findings from an empirical investigation conducted in West Germany are presented to support the theory that females drink heavily for different reasons than males. The underlying hypotheses are that: (1) female alcoholics learn different behavior patterns in childhood than male alcoholics, and (2) the development of heavy drinking among females is closely associated with marital and familial disturbances (including sexual difficulties and infidelity) rather than with occupational disturbances. Seven risk factors identified with female alcoholism are examined, and a 6-level chain of causative conditions of female drinking is developed. It is concluded that therapy for female alcoholism should be directed toward changing negative behavior patterns uniquely associated with the female personality as well as toward changing drinking behavior. Suggestions for treatment are offered. (NCALI)

205. Moskovic, S. Uticaj hronicnog trovanja alkoholom na ovarijumsku disfunckciju. [Effect of chronic alcohol intoxication on ovarian dysfunction.] *Srpski Arhiv za Celokupno Lekarstvo*, 1975, *103*, 751–758.

Data were collected from 321 chronic alcoholic women in Yugoslavia who attended the Outpatient Clinic of the Gynecological-Obstetrical Hospital in Belgrade, the VI Sanitarium in Belgrade, and the Women's Dispensary in Ljig. All subjects had been drinking regularly for at least 5 years, with 62.6% consuming between ½ to 1 liter of alcohol (typically brandy or cognac) daily. Chronic alcohol intoxication was found to be associated with cessation of ovarian function, regressive changes in the genital organs, a higher than average rate of early menopause, and a diminished sexual appetite.

206. Murphy, W. D., Coleman, E., Hoon, E., & Scott, C. Sexual dysfunction and treatment in alcoholic women. *Sexuality and Disability*, 1980, *3*, 240–255.

A total of 74 female inpatients at an alcoholic rehabilitation center and a halfway house were evaluated in terms of their sexual functioning. They were then given the opportunity to participate in a 12-session sexual enhancement program which addressed sex education, sexual awareness, sexual dysfunction, and sexual assertiveness. The subjects reported low levels of sexual activity: 23 of the 74 had not engaged in sexual intercourse in the past 6 months; 56 of 74 had never masturbated or had stopped masturbating. A large percent, 29.7%, reported little or no sexual desire; 28.4% reported inability to reach orgasm with a partner more than 50% of the time. Of those subjects who had been sexually active in the last 6 months, few reported experiencing sexual dysfunction. Overall, frequency of sexual problems among alcoholic women was no greater than that reported in a nonclinical sample. The authors believe that the alcoholic women minimized the extent of their sexual difficulties and that the data do not accurately represent the extent of sexual dysfunction among alcoholic women. Evidence for this appears in the discrepancies between some of the self-report measures and the sexual problems the women revealed in the later sessions of the sexual enhancement program that were not revealed during initial assessment. Participation in the sexual enhancement group was shown by the 23 participants effectively to increase satisfaction with existing relationships, communications, sexual arousability, and sexual knowledge.

207. Myerson, D. J. Clinical observations on a group of alcoholic prisoners, with special reference to women. *Quarterly Journal of Studies on Alcohol*, 1959, *20*, 555–572.

The primary aim of this paper is to paint a composite picture of the alcoholic prisoner with emphasis on commonalities in background and development. Conclusions are drawn from observations of incarcerated alcoholic prisoners participating in alcoholic rehabilitation programs in 2 Massachusetts correctional institutions. Three common features suggest a pattern: (1) a history of extreme and chronic deprivation in a traumatic setting, (2) prisoners show addictive-like food habits and prolonged bisexual relationships, and (3) by adolescence they lose whatever parental figures they have had or rebel with such vehemence as to make the home situation intolerable. Homosexual activities and incestuous sexual relationships began during latency and continued through adolescence. Adolescent struggles with sexuality lead to violent or dangerous acts and promiscuity. These features are found in both males and females but are most prominent in females.

208. Pinhas, V. L. An investigation to compare the degree to which alcoholic and non-alcoholic women report sex guilt and sexual control. (Doctoral dissertation, New York University, 1978). *Dissertation Abstracts International*, 1978, *39*, 7175A.

This study was designed to determine the degree to which alcoholic women in early sobriety report sex guilt and sexual control in comparison to a matched sample of nonalcoholic women. It was hypothesized that alcoholic women would report more sex guilt and less control over their sex lives than nonalcoholic women. Thirty-four alcoholic women with from 3 months to one year sobriety were drawn from alcoholism treatment facilities and/or Alcoholics Anonymous groups and matched on a number of demographic variables with 34 nonalcoholic women. Alcoholic women were found to report more sex guilt and less sexual control than nonalcoholic women. Other supplementary findings indicate a lower mean age for alcoholic women in comparison with past studies undertaken, perhaps indicating an increase in young women seeking assistance with alcoholism. (Author)

209. Pinhas, V. L. Sex guilt and sexual control in women alcoholics in early sobriety. *Sexuality and Disability*, 1980, *3*, 256–272.

This study was designed to determine the degree to which alcoholic women in early sobriety report sex guilt and sexual control in comparison to a matched sample of nonalcoholics. There were 34 women in each of the comparison groups. Alcoholic women reported significantly greater sex guilt and significantly less control over their sex lives than did nonalcoholic women. Implications for further investigation are discussed.

210. Potter, J. Women and sex—it's enough to drive them to drink! In V. Burtle (Ed.), *Women who drink, alcoholic experience and psychotherapy*. Springfield, IL: Charles C. Thomas, 1979.

The tendency for women to abuse alcohol is attributed to difficulties with intimacy, sex, and communication. The pain of their relationships with men drive women to drink, and some of the women who drink are alcoholics. The pain arises from the low self-esteem that is the result of childhood training. In addition, our culture offers the promise of happiness if we find the right person to love. Women and men are disappointed, pained, to discover that they are not able to bridge the gap between the sexes so that they may love and be loved. Responsibility for individuals' low self-esteem and problems with achieving intimacy are laid on our culture for raising males and females as different species. People whose intimacy needs are not met use alcohol to relieve the loneliness that compounds their problem. Counsellors are advised that alcohol may impair sexual function, or complicate an existing dysfunction, by its effect as a central nervous system depressant.

211. Rieth, E. Soziologische und psychologische ursachen der sucht bei frauen. [Sociological and psychological causes of addiction in women.] *Zeitschrift fuer Allgemeinmedizine,* 1971, *47,* 852–855.

Of 100 alcoholic women studied at a sanitarium in 1968–1969, 89 exhibited infantile behavior, 92 showed ego weakness, 60 found social contact difficult, 78 had a disturbed sexuality, 87 reported a negative attitude toward life, 72 reported a defect in family solidarity, 47 spoke of childhood insecurity, 70 came from over-protective homes, and 71 had a special position in their family. (NCALI)

212. Sandmaier, M. *The invisible alcoholics: Women and alcohol abuse in America.* New York: McGraw-Hill, 1980.

The history of social attitudes toward women's drinking is examined, and interviews with alcoholic women with various backgrounds are presented. The relation between drinking, drunkenness, and alcoholism and women's interest in or likelihood of having sex is discussed. Treatment services, referral and support centers, information services, and suggested readings are listed.

213. Schuckit, M. A. Sexual disturbance in the woman alcoholic. *Medical Aspects of Human Sexuality,* 1971, *6,* 44–65.

Promiscuity is observed in 5% of alcoholic women, while 95% complain of diminished interest in sex. Alcoholic women presenting prominent sexual adjustment problems can be grouped into 3 major categories, each with characteristic behavioral and sexual features. The sociopathic female alcoholic corresponds with the popular stereotype of the promiscuous drunken woman yet constitutes only 5% of alcoholic women. This group has a history of antisocial behavior prior to alcohol abuse, does not learn from previous behavior, and displays recklessness and disregard for the consequences of their behavior. Another type is the hysteric alcoholic. These women have many somatic complaints and find sex unpleasant, to be avoided whenever possible. The hysterical adjustment predates the alcoholism. The largest category consists of women for whom alcoholism is the first psychiatric problem to appear. These women tend to feel dissatisfied with sex and report difficulty achieving orgasm. Illustrative case histories are presented.

214. Schuckit, M. A., & Morrissey, E. R. Alcoholism in women: Some clinical and social perspectives with an emphasis on possible subtypes. In M. Greenblatt & M. A. Schuckit (Eds.), *Alcoholism problems in women and children.* New York: Grune & Stratton, 1976.

The goal of this chapter is to review what is known about alcoholism in women. Studies reveal that women alcoholics experience sexual adjustment problems; however, the type of sexual problems appears to be related to socioeconomic status. Studies with prisoners and low socioeconomic status groups find higher rates of promiscuity and involvement with prostitution among alcoholic women. These studies also find higher rates of homosexuality, as much as 20% among alcoholic female prisoners compared to reports of 0–10% among private female patients. Women in higher socioeconomic groups tend to report a lack of interest in sexual activity. Whether sexual difficulties are caused by heavy drinking and resulting relationship problems or were the causes of alcoholism cannot be determined.

215. Schuckit, M. A., & Morrissey, E. R. Psychiatric problems in women admitted to an alcoholic detoxification center. *American Journal of Psychiatry,* 1979, *136,* 611–617.

The psychiatric problems and demographic characteristics were compared in 5 diagnostic subgroups of women (N = 293) consecutively admitted to a public detoxification center. The primary diagnosis was alcoholism in 154, affective disorder in 40, antisocial personality (antisocial behavior before age 16) in 40, drug abuse in 18, and no diagnosis in 38. The mean ages were 45, 42, 30, and 33 years, respectively. Of the 154 primary alcoholics, most were Whites and of lower socioeconomic class, 48 were separated or divorced, 37% lived alone, 10% on skid row, and 19% were employed. They tended to drink daily and heavily (about 11 drinks per drinking day). The other groups had similar demographic characteristics. The prevalence of cirrhosis, excepting the no-diagnosis group, ranged from 22.1% to 29.3%. In the 5 diagnostic groups, 25–45% had a handicapped child, and 25–45% had had a miscarriage. The proportion of women in each diagnostic category who had engaged in sexual activity for money or for food or alcohol is reported. The most deviant groups in every respect were the drug abusers and those with antisocial personality. The latter had more problems with school, family, law, and drug use and were more likely than the primary alcoholics and the affective disorder groups (which resembled each other) to drink daily and to drink in bars and parks; they also used more alcohol substitutes, drank more, drank earlier in life, and had a greater incidence of personal psychiatric problems. It is concluded that female primary alcoholics seen in detoxification centers resemble more the primary male alcoholics seen in the same setting than they resemble middle-class female alcoholics. (RUCAS)

216. Shaw, S. The causes of increasing drinking problems amongst women: A general etiological theory. In Camberwell Council on Alcoholism, *Women and alcohol.* New York: Tavistock Publications, 1980.

Women have increasingly come to experience tension between established stereotypes and more flexible interpretations of appropriate sexual attitudes and behavior. It is in this area that studies have found the most acute identity problems of female problem drinkers. Sexual emancipation, like other aspects of emancipation, has served to increase the sex-role confusions, which has been found to precipitate drinking problems among women. Given (a) that problem drinking among women is triggered by sex-role problems and identity problems and (b) that problem drinking is highly concentrated among women who feel sexually inadequate and frigid, it is very likely that the changing climate of sexual mores has put more women at greater risk of turning to alcohol. (RUCAS)

217. Sheehan, M., & Watson, J. Response and recognition. In Camberwell Council on Alcoholism, *Women and alcohol*. New York: Tavistock Publications, 1980.

This chapter gives an overview of what are considered to be important factors in the treatment of women with alcohol problems. It includes a discussion of: (a) current services available in the United Kingdom and their suitability for women, (b) difficulties in women being detected at an early stage with their alcohol problems, and (c) indicators of drinking problems in women. The authors report that there is no evidence that drunken women are more promiscuous than drunken men. However, they go on to explain that it seems highly probable that the lowering of sexual inhibitions that occurs during intoxicated states will incur greater disapproval when it occurs in women than when it occurs in men. This, they believe, is due to the different standards of sexual morality that apply to men and women.

218. Topiar, A., & Satková, V. L. Sexuálni zivot alkoholicek. [Sexuality of female alcoholics.] *Protialkoholický Obzor*, 1976, *11*, 147–149.

This study analyzed the sex life of 22 women who abused alcohol for at least 5 years. More than half of the women were found to suffer damage to their sexuality. The damage included: disintegrated sexual behavior and decreased responsiveness and orgasmic capability. Forty percent of the married patients described the emotional ties to their husbands as impaired. The development of alcoholism was marked by development of parasitic and prostitute-like behavior that developed as family and coworker interpersonal conflicts increased.

219. Ullman, A. D. "Lady" drunks. In A. D. Ullman, *To know the difference*. New York: St. Martin's Press, 1960.

Alcoholism in women is automatically linked with sexual immorality. The female alcoholic is thought to be promiscuous or in danger of becoming so. She is more likely to feel the same way about sex as the male alcoholic: it interferes with drinking. Promiscuity, when it does occur, may be due to the woman's inability to resist exploitation, or she may exchange sexual favors for alcohol. This is a problem for a small number of alcoholic women and is different from truly promiscuous women who drink to excess to provide themselves with an excuse for having an affair.

220. Wilson, C. The family. In Camberwell Council on Alcoholism, *Women and alcohol*. New York: Tavistock Publications, 1980.

The theme of marital and sexual adjustment has figured quite prominently in the literature on alcoholic women. However, there is little information available regarding the effects of marital conflict on the family of the woman drinker. Research on alcoholic families has concentrated almost exclusively on male alcoholics and has failed to integrate findings from separate studies of the spouses and children and family interaction of problem drinkers. The lack of definitive information makes it difficult to derive firm strategies for the treatment of alcoholic women and their families. There are indications that involvement of the husband in treatment may be particularly important, especially where he, too, is a heavy drinker. (RUCAS)

221. Wood, H. P., & Duffy, E. L. Psychological factors in alcoholic women. *American Journal of Psychiatry*, 1966, *123*, 341–345.

Sixty-nine female alcoholics, who had been seen for alcoholism counseling and for whom adequate data exist, provide the foundation for generalizations about background features and subsequent adjustment of alcoholic women. These women were raised by cold, dominant mothers and passive fathers, some of whom were alcoholic. They were characterized as submissive, passively resentful, and lacking in a positive self-image. Their sex education was grossly inadequate. Most patients (88%) had married; however, the marriages tended to be emotionally unrewarding and sexual adjustment was poor. Often the husband introduced the wife to alcohol in order to release her sexual inhibitions. None of the patients reported homosexual experiences or problems, and none had ever been promiscuous.

3. Males

222. Aamark, C. A study in alcoholism: Clinical social-psychiatric and genetic investigations. *Acta Psychiatrica Scandanavica*, 1951 (Supplement 70), 1–283.

This study is aimed at evaluating the relative contributions of environment and heredity in the etiology of alcoholism. Subjects were 644 male patients in treatment for alcoholism at various Stockholm clinics, their parents, and their siblings. In this sample of alcoholics, impotence and sexual indifference were not as common as expected. Open homosexuality was rare. Venereal disease was more common among the alcoholics than "comparative material" (not defined; no comparison group was used in the study). Venereal disease infection occurred, on the average, prior to alcohol abuse. (RUCAS)

223. Akhtar, M. J. Sexual disorders in male alcoholics. In J. S. Madden, R. Walker, & W. H. Kenyon (Eds.), *Alcoholism and drug dependence*. New York: Plenum Press, 1977.

Data on age, social class (occupation), social stability, drinking history, and sexual functioning of 45 male, alcoholic inpatients, all previously or currently married, were collected through individual interviews, case records, and social reports. Information gathered from these sources indicates that alcoholism is associated, though not necessarily in a casual relationship, with sexual disorders in males, affecting libido, erection, and ejaculation. A relationship between length of alcohol abuse and severity of sexual disturbance was also revealed. (RUCAS)

224. Beaumont, G. Untoward effects of drugs on sexuality. In S. Crown (Ed.), *Psychosexual problems: Psychotherapy, counselling, and behavioral modification.* New York: Grune & Stratton, 1976.

Unwanted sexual effects have been observed in both males and females involved in drug therapy. Drugs may act adversely on sexual behavior both peripherally and centrally. They may affect sexuality by their action on endocrine pathways and hormonal secretions. Peripheral effects are usually brought about by drugs whose known pharmacological action is to alter or block biogenic amine-uptake mechanisms. Central effects of drugs on sexuality are thought to be brought about by their action on the limbic system and perhaps by hypothalamic endocrine disturbances. This chapter surveys what is known about the adverse effects of antihypertensive and psychotropic drugs on various aspects of sexual functioning in males and females. Mention is made of the impotence resulting from prolonged alcohol abuse which has been reported to persist for years after the achievement of sobriety.

225. Brajsa, P. Obiteljska patologija kod kronicnih alkoholicara. [Family pathology in chronic alcoholics.] *Alkoholizam, Beograd 8,* 1968, *2,* 32–49.

Of the 82 alcoholics treated at the mental hygiene clinic at Varazdin in Croatia, 47 had fathers, 43 had brothers, and 4 had mothers who were alcoholics. Twenty-five had suffered parental loss before age 15, and 38 had wives who need psychiatric help. Of the 101 children of these patients, 44 had neurotic and behavioral disturbances. Of 124 women with neurotic disturbances, the 40 whose husbands were alcoholics had a higher percentage of anxiety depressions (88% vs. 56%). Sexual incompatability and aggression and anxiety in their children were also more frequent in these women. A negative attitude toward the marriage of the parents among 450 school children was directly related to the frequency of drunkenness on the part of the father. (RUCAS)

226. Brzek, A. Muzská sexualita a alkohol. [Male sexuality and alcohol.] *Casopis Lékaru Ceskych,* 1979, *116,* 1024–1026.

Literature reviewed and the results of the author's own observations concerning the sexuality of alcoholics are referred to. Alcoholics show changes in hormonal relations affecting both androgens and gonadotropins. Responses to immediate alcohol ingestions vary. Abuse of alcohol makes for a deterioration of sexual functions in all components despite the fact that heterosexual development seems to be rather speeded up. Deviant behavior tends to develop even in subjects who have never suffered from deviation. There are strikingly poor spermatological findings, even when compared with a control group of impotent men. (English abstract and English title were provided as a summary at the beginning of foreign article cited above.) (Author)

227. Brzek, A., Raboch, J., & Lachman, M. Der sexuelle status des alkoholikers. [The sexual status of alcoholics.] *Sexualmedizin,* 1977, *6,* 478–480.

A comparison of the questionnaire studies of 104 alcoholics seeking treatment and 101 normospermic and sexually potent male controls disclosed, among other things, significant differences in male sexual function (SFM according to Mellan) in the following respects: alcoholics have a lesser degree of sexual desire; with them, the number of sexual contacts as well as the frequency of coitus and orgasm are smaller; and their erection is of a lesser quality. Another study on the course of heterosexual maturation, covering 141 alcoholics and 112 normal males, showed that alcoholics had an accelerated development and that the reduction of sexual capacity in them only sets in gradually in the course of their alcohol misuse. (English abstract was provided as a summary at the beginning of foreign article cited above.) (Author)

228. Brzek, A., & Skála, J. Sexuální funkce alkoholiku. [Sexual functions of alcoholics.] *Protialkoholický Obzor,* 1976, *11,* 129–132.

Sexual function was measured in 104 alcoholics using Mellan's SFM questionnaire. The questionnaire measures 10 components of sexual functioning: sexual appetite, frequency of sexual satiation without intercourse, frequency of sexual intercourse, frequency of effecting intercourse, erectile functioning, duration of intercourse, disposition before intercourse, satisfaction after intercourse, feelings of success in sexual life, and occurrence of dysfunction. Results were compared to a control group revealing subnormal values more frequently among the alcoholics. With the exception of the duration of intercourse, the differences were statistically significant. The difference in feelings of satisfaction after sexual intercourse proved most significant. (English abstract and English title were provided as a summary at the end of foreign article cited above.) (Author)

229. Burton, G., & Kaplan, H. M. Sexual behavior and adjustment of married alcoholics. *Quarterly Journal of Studies on Alcohol,* 1968, *29,* 603–609.

The sexual behavior and interaction of alcoholic husbands and their wives are studied, and the degree of their agreement on sexual attitudes and practices is determined. A questionnaire on sexual behavior and adjustment was administered to 16 married couples of whom the husbands were alcoholics, and 16 couples without alcohol problems. Both groups were receiving counseling for marital difficulties. Some of the findings are as follows: the alcoholic husbands reported sexual intercourse 1.6 times a week, their wives 2.1 times; 7 of the husbands and 10 of the wives were satisfied by this frequency. Many wives reported withholding sexual activity in order to control their husbands' drinking. The alcoholics' wives experienced sexual orgasm "nearly always" and more frequently than did the wives of the nonalcoholics. The alcoholics and their wives were able to discuss sexual matters more freely than the nonalcoholic couples. Most of the alcoholics (81%) and their wives (63%) reported that the husband took the initiative in sexual activity. Both alcoholics and their wives reported some disagreement over sexual adjustment, but considerably less than the nonalcoholic couples. While 62% of the alcoholic couples' comments about dissatisfaction were over attitudes, 67% of the nonalcoholic couples' comments were over techniques; the difference is attributed to the alcoholic couples' greater ability to discuss sexual matters. (RUCAS)

230. Butler, R. N. Sexual advice to the aging male. *Medical Aspects of Human Sexuality*, 1975, *9*, 155–156.

Sexual problems in the elderly are discussed in this article, and some specific suggestions for office counseling are given. Common causes of loss of sex drive in later years may include depression, anxiety, boredom, fear of heart attack, alcohol abuse, antidepressants, tranquilizers, poor physical fitness, obesity, and diabetes. (Author)

231. Chiles, J. A., Stauss, F. S., & Benjamin, L. S. Marital conflict and sexual dysfunction in alcoholic and non-alcoholic couples. *British Journal of Psychiatry*, 1980, *137*, 266–273.

Marital interaction appears to be relevant to alcoholism. This study compares 2 groups of couples, each presenting with sexual dysfunction. One group has an alcoholic member in each couple, one group does not. The presenting sexual complaint in the alcoholic couples was impotence, with concomitant frigidity in 2 cases. Data are presented suggesting that alcoholic marriages can be distinguished, in a clinically useful way, from other troubled marriages. Alcoholic husbands feel submissive but are not being forced by their wives to be so. This suggests a therapeutic approach different from the one that would be taken if the wives were actually dominating. No specific data on the sexual aspects of the couples are presented. (Author)

232. Cobb, J. Morbid jealousy. *British Journal of Hospital Medicine*, 1979, *21*, 511; 513–514; 516–518.

The underlying psychopathology, the interpersonal factors, and the management of morbid jealousy are discussed. As early as 1847 Marcel stated that delusions of jealousy were generally met in alcoholics. Kraft-Ebing claimed that about 80% of male alcoholics who still had sexual relations were afflicted by delusions of jealousy. Kolle identified 3 subgroups: jealous drunkards, exogenous drunkards, and delusional drinkers (paranoid jealousy). The first group includes jealous, inadequate men who had become jealous drunkards. The second group includes persons with alcoholic hallucinosis, and the third group includes schizophrenics. More recent research has shown that while alcohol frequently inflames preexisting symptoms and precipitates violence, it is only rarely a primary cause of morbid jealousy. Alcohol may thus be more of forensic than etiological importance. (RUCAS)

233. Cohen, D. C., & Krause, M. S. *Casework with the wives of alcoholics*. New York: Family Service Association of America, 1971. (Cited in T. J. Paolino, & B. S. McCrady *The alcoholic marriage: Alternative perspectives*. New York: Grune & Stratton, 1977, 120.)

A total of 298 cases involving an alcohol-abuse problem were assigned to one of 2 treatment groups. In one group, treatment was based on the disease concept of alcoholism; the other group of caseworkers used a "traditional" approach in which the alcoholism was viewed as a symptom of family problems. Follow-up data, obtained at least 6 months

after the end of treatment, and based on interviews with the nonalcoholic wives, suggested a greater decrease in drinking in the disease-oriented group than in the traditional group. In the intact marriages (30% of both groups were separated at follow-up), however, the wives treated by the traditional workers reported more sexual satisfaction, more satisfaction with their husbands as husbands and fathers, and fewer employment problems. It would appear that wives reported improvement in the areas focused on in treatment (alcoholism in the disease approach; marital conflicts in the traditional approach) and that changes in the 2 areas (drinking and general satisfaction) were relatively independent. (Author)

234. Cohen, S. Drugs and sexuality. In S. Cohen, *The substance abuse problems* (Vol. 13). New York: Haworth Press, 1981.

Alcohol may provoke sexual desires but adversely affect sexual performance. Male alcoholics often complain of impotence and its frustrations. Over a long period of drinking, metabolism of the gonadal hormones is deranged. Plasma testosterone levels are lowered by substantial alcohol intake. Testicular atrophy and gynecomastia can result from a combination of low testosterone levels from reduced production, and high leuteinizing hormone levels from impaired metabolism in the damaged liver. (RUCAS)

235. DeMoya, D., & DeMoya, A. Alcohol and impotence. *RN Magazine*, 1980, *43*, 88.

The authors respond to a reader question about alcohol's effect on erection in the question and answer section of this magazine. Causes and therapy for impotence due to alcohol are briefly discussed. (RUCAS)

236. Deniker, P., de Saugy, D., & Ropert, M. The alcoholic and his wife. *Comprehensive Psychiatry*, 1964, *5*, 374–383.

In this study conducted by the Clinique des Maladies Mentales et de l'Encéphale in Paris, 3 groups of couples were compared: Psychiatric Alcoholics (PA), alcoholics with chronic, severe character or behavior disorders; Digestive Alcoholics, those with chronic hepato-digestive disorders such as cirrhosis and chronic gastritis; and Controls, a matched group of nonalcoholic, nonpsychiatric patients whose disorders required hospitalization, such as fractures and arthritis. Subjects were recruited from several hospitals and outpatient clinics in Paris. Interviews with the alcoholic couples revealed low frequency of sexual activity at the time of the addiction and earlier in married life, before the onset of alcoholism, markedly less than the controls. Wives of the alcoholics differed from controls in that many were frigid from the beginning of marriage, especially in the PA group.

237. Drew, L. R. H., Moon, J. R., Buchanan, F. H., & Thomas, B. B. Counselling the family of the alcoholic. *Australian Journal of Alcoholism and Drug Dependence*, 1974, *1*, 76–78.

Attention is drawn to the fact that alcoholism is a family illness and, properly, the responsibility of the family doctor. Family counselling is an important area of preventive medicine. Family members need to understand how they contribute to perpetuating alcoholism and how they may help in recovery. They need help to deal realistically with day-to-day occurrences while drinking continues or to face the need for separation. Once an alcoholic begins to recover, new problems arise which may more seriously threaten the family than active alcoholism. Even after recovery, problems such as depression, delinquency and sexual disinterest will be present and will need the doctor's expert attention in their resolution. The relationship between sex and alcoholism in the male is described. Counselling of the families of alcoholics is a very important community responsibility of every family physician.

238. Fedetov, D. D., Model, K. S., & Zhukov, Yu. T. *Referativnyi Zhurnal. Farmakologiva. Khimioterapevticheskiye Sredstva.* [Sexual disturbances in patients with chronic alcoholism as a complication following disulfiram treatment.] *Toksikologiya,* 1969, *7,* 876.

Examination results are given for 15 chronic alcoholic patients who had suffered from alcoholism for an average of 15.4 years. These patients complained of sexual problems and demonstrated sexual weakness after taking disulfiram. (NCALI)

239. Felstein, I. The organic causes of impotence. *British Journal of Sexual Medicine,* 1973, *1,* 33–37.

Contending with organic illness can be complicated by concomitant impotence. Infection, bone fracture, congenital defects, and medication can interfere with neurological or endocrine systems and undermine sexual performance. Misuse of morphine and addictive drugs, including alcohol, may affect potency as a result of personality deterioration and depression or distortion of libido.

240. Freedberg, E. J., & Johnston, W. E. Outcome with alcoholics seeking treatment voluntarily or after confrontation by their employer. *Journal of Occupational Medicine,* 1980, *22,* 83–86.

Treatment results with 370 alcoholics (95% male) who sought treatment after being threatened with dismissal by their employers were compared with results with 58 alcoholics who sought treatment voluntarily. Data indicated that voluntary clients were experiencing significantly greater problems in a wide range of psychosocial areas when they entered treatment than were mandatory clients, whereas mandatory clients had a poorer work record in terms of productivity and of drinking behavior interfering with work. After treatment, however, there were few differences between the groups in terms of psychosocial behavior, work performance, and drinking behavior. The only differences between the 2 groups at one-year follow-up were that the mandatory group had scores showing significantly better functioning than the voluntary group on the overassertion and marital sex subscales of the Ontario Problem Assessment Battery. The results suggest that coercion is a useful tool in inducing alcoholics to seek treatment, since outcome with mandatory clients is similar to that with voluntary clients and since it is likely that few of the mandatory clients would have

sought treatment without pressure from their employers. (Author)

241. Goodwin, D. W., Crane, J. B., & Guze, S. B. Felons who drink: An 8-year follow-up. *Quarterly Journal of Studies on Alcohol,* 1971, *32,* 136–147.

In an 8-year follow-up study of 223 convicted male felons previously studied, 176 were available for interview. Of these, 118 were diagnosed as alcoholics or problem drinkers. Analysis of 360 variables obtained at original and follow-up interviews revealed the alcoholics to have significantly higher proportions of various problems and characteristics including: multiple sex partners, homosexuality, and impotence for nearly a quarter of the alcoholics (no nonalcoholics).

242. Gross, W. F., Carpenter, L. L., & Alder, L. O. Problems of adjustment reported by alcoholics prior to leaving a hospital treatment program. *Quarterly Journal of Studies on Alcohol,* 1971, *32,* 454–456.

The Mooney Problem Check List was administered to 53 male alcoholics (mean age, 42.5 years; mean years of schooling, 10.6) after completion of the 6th of 8 weeks of intensive treatment at the Lexington (KY) Veterans Administration Hospital. The 2 categories with the highest percentage of items checked were self-improvement and economic security (17% and 15% of 1,908 items). Of the 15 items most frequently checked, 7 were in the personality category. The importance of a program aimed at alcoholics' specific concerns as they near completion of treatment—economic insecurity, poor sex relations, and emotional instability—is discussed. (RUCAS)

243. Henc, I. Alkoholizam-ljubomora i smetnje potencije. [Jealousy of alcoholics and disturbances of potency.] *Anali Bolnice Dr. M. Stojanovic,* 1967, *6,* 261–265.

Manifestations of jealousy and the disturbances of sexual potency were studied in chronic alcoholics by prolonged observation of the patients and study of their domestic environment. The results confirm an etiologic dependence of the mental and functional phenomena upon alcohol consumption. (Author)

244. Horowitz, J. D., & Goble, A. J. Drugs and impaired male sexual function. *Drugs,* 1979, *18,* 206–217.

This review examines male sexual dysfunction resulting from drug use. Drugs affect sex through effects on the nervous system, the cardiovascular system, and the endocrine system. Reports of male sexual dysfunction call for a complete physical examination to rule out organic causes such as diabetes mellitus and alcoholism. Use of prescription and nonprescription drugs can have side-effects resulting in impotence. The effects of commonly used drugs, including alcohol, are described.

245. Jensen, S. B. Seksualvaner og seksuelle problemer hos alkoholister: En undersogelse af 100 mandlige alkoholister mellem 30 og 45 ar. [Sexual habits and sexual problems among alcohol addicts: Report of an investigation of 100 male alcoholics between 30 and 45 years.] *Ugeskrift for Laeger*, 1977, *139*, 35–40.

One hundred male alcoholics aged 30–45 years who had been treated with disulfiram (Antabuse) for 4–8 weeks were consecutively questioned about their sexual habits and problems. The object of this investigation was to obtain background material that could form the basis of improved sexual advice for these patients. A combined questionnaire and interview technique was employed. Histories of early sexual activity were found to be unconnected with present sexual difficulties and onset of alcoholism. Of the men questioned, 63% had sexual difficulties primarily in the form of reduced libido and impotence. Two-thirds experienced this dysfunction in relation to the commencement of treatment for alcoholism. No change in quantitative sexuality occurred in this connection as judged by frequency of coitus, and this was found to be within the normal range of variation. Sixteen percent of the patients had not had coitus during the period of investigation. No connection could be found between the occurrence of sexual difficulties and the duration of alcoholism or the present partnership. The direct neurotoxic effects of alcohol or disulfiram therapy were found to be of limited significance but the psychological reaction at the commencement of treatment for the addiction appears to be of considerable significance, and treatment must primarily be directed toward this. (English abstract and English title were provided as a summary at the end of foreign article cited above.) (Author)

246. Jensen, S. B. Sexual customs and dysfunction in alcoholics: Part I. *British Journal of Sexual Medicine*, 1979, *6*, 29–32.

One hundred male alcoholics, 30–45 years of age, who had received outpatient treatment for 4 to 8 weeks including disulfiram (Antabuse) were interviewed about their sexual customs and sexual dysfunctions. The study was conducted by a combined questionnaire and interview technique. It is concluded that the sexual dysfunction of alcoholic men in most cases seems to have psychological-interpersonal causes, giving the possibility of combining common alcoholism therapy with modern sex therapy. (Author)

247. Jensen, S. B. Sexual customs and dysfunction in alcoholics: Part II. *British Journal of Sexual Medicine*, 1979, *6*, 30–34.

Sexual problems are common among male alcoholics, as was made evident by 63% of the patients in this study complaining of sexual dysfunction. The most common symptoms were impotence and reduced libido. Nearly two-thirds of the patients felt that their sexual dysfunction originated just at the beginning of the alcoholism treatment. However, in this regard no change in sexual intercourse frequency the month before and after this event could be demonstrated. The alcoholic man seems to experience a qualitative, but not quantitative change in his sexuality. The demonstration that the duration of alcoholism was not related to the occurrence of sexual dysfunction weakens the hypothesis that this dys-

function is due to neuropathy; neither does the disulfiram medication seem to be the reason for sexual complaints, as reported in an earlier study. The sexual problems of alcoholics have their roots mostly in psychological and interpersonal relations which include some of the following factors: (a) a basic personality structure including a low self-esteem of mind and body, (b) a role of feeling chronically tired without a capacity for sexual activity, (c) middle-aged single men with weak interpersonal contacts, (d) an acute complex of problems resulting from the abrupt change from daily heavy drinking to total abstinence, (e) changes in the partner relationship, the power balance being disturbed, (f) a "loser" group within society, and (g) drugs, alcoholic dementia, and neuropathy. Establishing that the sexual dysfunctions of alcoholics in most cases may have a psychological etiology, we feel that sex therapy for alcoholic couples might be able to aid existing alcoholism therapy. (Author)

248. Jensen, S. B. Sexual dysfunction in male diabetics and alcoholics: A comparative study. *Sexuality and Disability*, 1981, *4*, 215–219.

Sexual dysfunction was evaluated in 3 groups of males 30–45 years of age: 52 diabetics, 48 alcoholics, and 30 men from a general practice. Diabetics and alcoholics showed the same incidence and symptom pattern of sexual dysfunction, both groups differed significantly from the controls in symptom patterns and in incidence of sexual dysfunction. This difference consisted of a higher rate of erectile dysfunction and reduced libido. Premature ejaculation was the most common symptom in the control group. Sexual dysfunction was uncorrelated to duration of diabetes and alcohol addiction. Diabetic sexual dysfunction was overrepresented among patients having peripheral neuropathy, although 52% of diabetics reporting sexual dysfunction were without signs of neuropathy. The results may be explained partly by neurological damage as well as by problems concerning life quality of chronically ill patients. We suggest a more active communication about lifestyle including the sexual subaspects. This communication should be based on a better knowledge from more stringent studies of relationships of sexual dysfunction and somatic disease. (Author)

249. Johnson, J. H., & Harris, W. G. Personality and behavioral characteristics related to divorce in a population of male applicants for psychiatric evaluation. *Journal of Abnormal Psychology*, 1980, *89*, 510–513.

A replicated correlational study is reported in which a comprehensive pool of items pertaining to psychopathology, personality, social history, and medical history are related to the married/divorced distinction in a sample of applicants for psychiatric evaluation. A few significant correlations are obtained. Results indicate that there are few enduring personality characteristics related to divorce. Those found suggest that divorced males have lesser ego controls than those who sustain marriage. Divorced subjects endorsed items that suggest impaired social/sexual functioning, a tendency toward alcohol abuse, and relatively unconventional beliefs. (Author)

250. Jones, H. B., & Jones, H. C. *Sensual drugs: Deprivation and rehabilitation of the mind.* Cambridge, MA: Cambridge University, 1977, 131–132.

Alcohol, like barbiturates and tranquilizers, is a nervous system depressant. It may induce sensations that increase sexual desire while dulling the mind and impairing coordination. It primarily releases inhibition, rarely enhances sex, and produces loss of ability with high doses. Chronic alcohol use can lead to impotence and damaged testes. Loss of interest in sex may result from the alcoholic's acceptance of alcohol as a substitute for sex and from diminished physical vitality.

251. Karacan, I., Snyder, S., Salis, P. J., Williams, R. L., & Derman, S. Sexual dysfunction in male alcoholics and its objective evaluation. In W. E. Fann, I. Karacan, A. D. Pokorny, & R. L. Williams (eds.), *Phenomenology and treatment of alcoholism.* New York: Spectrum Publications, 1980.

Two groups of 6 men underwent monitoring of nocturnal penile tumescence (NPT) for 3 consecutive nights. One group consisted of impotent male patients being evaluated for radical treatment of impotence, i.e., implantation of penile prosthesis. During the course of evaluation, it was concluded that the patients had histories of significant alcohol abuse or misuse. The other 6 were healthy controls matched for age. Comparisons between the groups revealed that they obtained equal amounts of sleep, and that minutes of NPT were not significantly different. However, when NPT comparisons were examined more closely, the alcoholic impotent group displayed significantly less full NPT in terms of number of full NPT episodes and the total number of minutes of full NPT than did controls. Also, the impotent group displayed a greater number of partial NPT episodes than did controls. The authors compare these findings with a similar study using impotent diabetics and tentatively conclude that diabetics may have more organic involvement than impotent alcoholics. They point out the need for more research into the physiological and psychological mechanism involved in erectile dysfunction.

252. Khodakov, N. M., & Martynov, V. V. O zavisimosti seksual'nykh rasstroisty pri alkogolizme ot polovoi konstitutsii. [Do development or non-development of potency disturbances in alcoholic disease depend on sexual constitution?] In A. A. Portnoy (Ed.), *Problems of contemporary sexopathology.* Moscow: Ministry of Public Health of the RSFSR, 1972.

The first experience in application of some criteria from the vector scale for evaluation of male sexual constitution shows that of 2 statistically comparable groups of alcoholic patients potency disturbances developed more frequently and were more manifest in the group belonging to a weak variety. (English abstract and English title were provided as a summary at the end of foreign article cited above.) (Author)

253. Lamache, A., Davost, H., Chuberre, & Delalande. L'activité génésique des alcooliques chroniques.

[Sexual functioning of chronic alcoholics.] *Bulletin de L'Academie Nationale de Medecine,* 1952, *136,* 530–532.

A report on 143 male alcoholics, aged 28–45; "their intoxication" was due in two-thirds of the cases to cider and cider brandy, in one-third to wine and aperitifs. No cirrhosis or polyneuritis was included in the sample. Only 12 complained spontaneously about sexual disorders (and in those it was probably the wife who prompted them to complain). Yet it was found that 10% of the group had lost all desire for sex; 41% were capable only of episodic and imperfect acts; 32% continued to be attracted to the opposite sex but were unable to perform satisfactorily; 17% were impotent; 120 had small, soft and hyposensitive testicles; 98 had scant body hair; 56 had feminine hair distribution; 3 had gynecomastia. It is concluded that the alcoholic becomes uninterested in all things, including sex; his egotism grows; he becomes prematurely senile. (RUCAS)

254. Lemere, F., & Smith, J. W. Alcohol-induced sexual impotence. *American Journal of Psychiatry,* 1973, *130,* 212–213.

The authors contend that alcohol-induced sexual impotence is neurogenic in nature and often irreversible. They note that impotence resulting from prolonged alcohol abuse may persist even after years of sobriety. The problem is regarded as neither a psychological nor a hormonal defect, but rather as due to the destructive effect of alcohol on the neurogenic reflex arc that serves the process of erection. That the damage is irreversible would account for the inability of some men to reattain potency. Heavy drinkers experiencing early signs of sexual failure are advised to stop drinking in the hope that sobriety and time will restore their sexual vigor. (RUCAS)

255. Mello, N. K. Alcoholism and the behavioral pharmacology of alcohol: 1967–1977. In M. A. Lipton, A. DiMascio, & K. F. Killam (Eds.), *Psychopharmacology: A generation of progress.* New York: Raven Press, 1978.

This chapter contains a detailed overview of important issues in alcohol and alcoholism research. The chapter is divided into 2 parts: alcohol use and abuse and behavioral effects of alcohol. Relevant recent research, done primarily with males, is discussed. A portion of the section on behavioral effects of alcohol is devoted to alcohol's effect on sexuality. Observations from the studies reviewed are: sexual function in alcoholics may be impaired due to disruption of gonadal functioning; sexual arousal is attenuated with alcohol ingestion, the effects increasing with increasing amounts of alcohol; the primary effect of alcohol is to raise the threshold for both erective and ejaculatory reflexes; and even low doses of alcohol interfere with the erectile response.

256. Morin, R. A. Alcoholic man—Two much/too little. *Journal of Psychedelic Drugs,* 1980, *12,* 167–169.

The author contends that, when alcohol and alcoholism cause impotence and disinterest in sex, the alcoholic fails to blame the chemical or chemicals that previously were known to enhance his sexuality. Instead of blaming alcohol, he begins to question his own sexual identity or his own physical health and is very likely to go out in search of more potent and effective erotic stimuli to overcome his impotence. The following spheres of life that control sexuality and that are influenced by alcohol are briefly discussed: (1) organic changes in the body which physically interfere with the male alcoholic's sex life and (2) the modified male alcoholic's sexual identity. It is concluded that the chemicals the male alcoholic or drug abuser is consuming are the most likely cause of any sexual dysfunction and that recovery may be as simple as becoming abstinent. (NCALI)

257. Naess, K. Impotens fremkalt av medikamenter. [Impotence caused by drugs.] *Tidsskrift for Den norske laegeforening nr,* 1977, *97,* 468–469.

Alcohol, as well as a variety of drugs including disulfiram, may cause impotence. Disulfiram prevents the synthesis of norepinephrine, and this may not only disturb the sexual functions, but also cause the depression and fatigue often seen in patients under disulfiram treatment. (RUCAS)

258. Neshkov, N. S. Sostoyaniye spermatogeneza i polovoi funktsii u zloupotreblyayushchikh alkogolem. [The state of spermatogenesis and sexual function in those who abuse alcohol.] *Urachebnoe Delo,* 1969, *2,* 130–131.

Among the male patients of a sexological institute in the Lugansk district seen in the last 4 years, 76 were found to have drunk alcohol to excess for 5 to 11 years. The sexual abnormalities included weak erections (20 patients), premature ejaculations (in 25), and a combination of these (in 24). The ejaculate was less than normal in volume in 63, and abnormally viscous in 58. Some inactive spermatozoa were found in 12 and some morphological changes in spermatozoa in 13. Careful study of each patient disclosed no other possible causative factors in their anamnesis than drinking. Prolonged frequent use of alcohol may lead to dysfunction of sexual glands and changes in the excretory and androgenic functions. (RUCAS)

259. Orford, J., Guthrie, S., Nicholls, P., Oppenheimer, E., Egert, S., & Hensman, C. Self-reported coping behavior of wives of alcoholics and its association with drinking outcome. *Journal of Studies on Alcohol,* 1975, *36,* 1254–1267.

One hundred women whose husbands were counselled or treated because of their excessive drinking completed a shortened version of the Orford-Guthrie questionnaire (a measure of "coping with drinking"). Each family was subjected to follow-up 12 months after the initial consultation, and the association between the coping behavior reported at the initial consultation and the drinking reported at the follow-up was analyzed. High-frequency coping behavior appears to be associated with a relatively poor outcome, whatever the precise nature of the coping behavior employed. The coping components whose items are most uniformly associated with a relatively poor prognosis are those that suggest withdrawal or disengagement from the marital bond, such as the wife's withdrawal from sexual activity. Elements showing a higher degree of involvement such as pleading, arguing, hitting, jealousy, ridicule, or disposing of alcohol are not associated with a poor outcome.

260. Paige, P. E., LaPointe, W., & Krueger, A. The marital dyad as a diagnostic and treatment variable in alcohol addiction. *Psychology,* 1971, *8,* 54–73.

The Minnesota Multiphasic Personality Inventory (MMPI) was given to 25 women whose husbands were treated for alcoholism at Pioneer Foundation, Pomona, CA, and their scores were compared with those of their husbands on the 13 basic MMPI scales and on 40 selected subscales. The scores of the wives indicated hyperactivity, lack of personal conscience development, denial of dependency anxiety, and self-alienation. The feminine-interest scores indicated sexual problems. The often noted martyr complex was not seen. The husbands were characterized by depression, lack of activity, social alienation, self-alienation, and denial of dependency anxiety and tended to be physically and mentally tired. The masculine-interest scores indicated sexual problems. Maladaptive marital relationships were evident. While both partners need contact and excitement, they are unable to obtain satisfaction directly because of their mutual defense mechanisms. They both show passive, withdrawn behavior and a "suspicious feminine" nature. The neurotic tendencies of both spouses make for the basic discordance in their marriage. Treatment and rehabilitation must take into consideration: (1) the partners' inability to satisfy each other's needs in an adaptive way and (2) the fact that the wives have a vested interest in the maladaptation and that they perceive change in the relationship as disruptive and crisis provoking.

261. Paredes, A. Marital-sexual factors in alcoholism. *Medical Aspects of Human Sexuality,* 1973, *7,* 98–115.

The effect of alcoholism on marital and sexual relations is discussed. It is stated that in middle-aged men impotence is associated more often with the excessive use of alcohol than with any other factor. The subordination of sexual gratification to drinking is noted as a commonplace of the alcoholic individual.

262. Piron, E. Assessment of the male alcoholic's response to women through the use of visual stimuli. (Doctoral dissertation, Loyola University of Chicago, 1975). *Dissertation Abstracts International,* 1975, *36,* 454B–455B. (University Microfilms No. 75-14,523)

Personality characteristics of dependence, ambivalence, immature sexuality, and narcissism, frequently associated in the literature with alcoholism, suggest that alcoholics' relationships with women are observably different from nonalcoholics. This investigation explores the male alcoholic's attitude toward women by assessing his preferences for pictures representing women in 4 roles or images: motherly, nurturant, or protective; erotic or seductive; mature, with no reference to the first 2 roles; and immature or adolescent. There are 3 groups of 24 subjects: alcoholics, schizophrenics, and normal controls. The schizophrenic group showed a greater preference for the sexual pictures than did the alcoholics or normals, both of whom preferred the adolescent pictures. Lowest preference was for the motherly pictures with the schizophrenics showing the strongest lack of preferences. Lack of differentiation between the alcoholics and normals may be due to a social desirability artifact which resulted from alcoholics and normals both putting their "best foot" forward. Furthermore, within the alcoholic group there were a number of different personality types which, when combined, cancelled out differences from the normal controls.

263. Powell, B. J., Viamontes, J. A., & Brown, C. S. Alcohol effects on the sexual potency of alcoholic and non-alcoholic males. *Sexuality,* 1974, *10,* 78–80.

The effect of alcohol on sexual potency was investigated through interviews of 50 alcoholic males and 20 nonalcoholic males. Subjects reported on their ability to become erect when intoxicated and when sober. Alcohol was found to impair general sexual performance, and particularly the ability to ejaculate. Overall, it was found that the effects of alcohol on sexual potency were transient. The research points up the need for more systematic studies in this area. (RUCAS)

264. Renshaw, D. C. Impotence in diabetics. In J. LoPiccolo & L. LoPiccolo (Eds.), *Handbook of sex therapy.* New York: Plenum Press, 1978.

Among men who have had diabetes for over 6 years, 48% may be impotent. The impotence is usually interpreted by patient and physician as a complication of the disease. A diagnosis of organic impotence may be premature. The author reports that in working with diabetic males other factors have been found to play a role in the etiology of impotence. These are: alcohol abuse, anxiety, depression, and anger. When these factors are dealt with, impotence may be relieved. The author recommends carefully screening for these factors before recommending a penile prosthesis. Three case histories describe successful sex therapy with alcohol-abusing diabetics and their wives.

265. Sexual function loss tied to alcohol abuse. *Public Health Reports,* 1980, *95,* 497–498.

Research dealing with male sexual dysfunction as a result of alcohol abuse is described in this brief article. Studies conducted at the General Clinical Research Center of the Presbyterian University Hospital in Pittsburgh have shown that drinking enough alcohol to cause a hangover can decrease testosterone levels in normal, healthy men who may only be occasional drinkers. Symptoms of alcohol abuse have been found in many young men complaining of infertility. (NCALI)

266. Sidman, J. M. Sexual functioning and the physically disabled adult. *The American Journal of Occupational Therapy,* 1977, *31,* 81–85.

A person's sexual readjustment following a physical disability has traditionally been ignored by health care professionals. Since the occupational therapist often facilitates a person's resumption of activities of daily living, the therapist is in a special position to provide counselling. Understanding, support, and correct information are needed most. As derived from a search of the literature, sexual functioning is discussed in relation to the following disabilities: stroke, heart disease, diabetes mellitus, muscular dystrophy, multiple sclerosis, renal disease, spinal cord injury, pulmonary disease, arthritis, and alcoholism. Alcohol-induced impotence may persist after years of sobriety. Chronic abuse can lead to damage to neurologic reflex arc subserving erection, gonadal failure, and hypothalamic-pituitary supression. There are reports that Antabuse, a drug used in the management of alcoholic patients, may contribute to impotence. (Author)

267. Smith, J. W., Lemere, F., & Dunn, R. B. Impotence in alcoholism. *Northwest Medicine,* 1972, *71,* 523–524.

The authors found that over the past 35 years approximately 8% of over 17,000 male alcoholic people had experienced impotence after detoxification. Gradually, 50% of those returned to their previous level of competence, 25% remained relatively impotent, and 25% suffered absolute impotence. One possible explanation given for this phenomenon concerns alcohol-induced damage to structures involved in sexual function. It is observed that although alcohol may temporarily stimulate sexual ability, it can undermine sexual potency in the long run. (RUCAS)

268. Stankusev, T., Protic, M., & Shishkov, A. [Sexual troubles in alcoholics.] *Neurologiya Psikhiatriya i Neurokhirurgiya,* 1974, *13,* 409–415.

Clinical studies were carried out on the sexual dynamics of 373 male alcoholics aged from 20 to 50 years. Sexual problems were found in 51%. The longer the abuse of alcoholic drink, the higher the percentage of sexual problems. Most patients showed disturbances of the 4 components of intercourse: libido, erection, ejaculation, and orgasm. Such problems were most frequent in drinkers of spirits. Significant changes in the fertility functions were established: reduction of the ejaculate, reduction in number and motility of spermatozoa, and a higher percentage of pathological forms. Increased zincuria in the ejaculate, lower levels of luteinizing hormone (LH) and follicle-stimulating hormone (FSH), reduced LH/FSH ratio, and disturbed spermatogenic activity were also found. (English abstract and English title were provided as a summary at the end of foreign article cited above.) (Author)

269. Student, V., & Matova, A. Vyoj psychickych poruch u manzelek alkoholiku. [The development of psychic disorders in wives of alcoholics.] *Ceskoslovenska Psychiatrie,* 1969, *65,* 23–29.

Of 40 wives of hospitalized alcoholics, 35 complained of psychological disturbances developed during marriage. A protracted anxiety-depressive neurosis was found in 17 women, 8 suffered from reactive depressions, 6 from the neurasthenic syndrome, and 4 from repeated depressive reactions. Psychosomatic diseases were also frequent. The disorders became manifest usually after several years of married life, particularly at the time when attempts to change the husband's drinking habits having failed, the woman became resigned to her fate. The intensity of the disturbances was roughly proportional to the degree of the husband's misbehavior with respect to family and sexual life; 75% of the women suffered from mistreatment; 40% had an aversion to sexual intercourse. The personality deviations of the wives included immaturity, dependency, and feelings of inferiority based apparently on disrupted family conditions found in the childhood of 65% of the women. This and other conditions (12 were divorced, 7 pregnant before marriage) played a role in the inconsiderate choice of husbands and in the ambivalent attitudes of the women. (RUCAS)

270. Terent'yev, Ye.I. K probleme seksual'noi patologii pri alkogol'nom brede revnosti. [Sexual pathology in alcoholic delusions of jealousy.] *Zhurnal Nevropatologii*, 1978, *78*, 1705–1710.

The data on sex pathology in alcoholic delusions of jealousy with sadomasochist behavior are reported. Such behavior was seen when the patients tried to force their wives to acknowledge infidelity. A total of 196 patients were studied. Abnormal behavior was characterized by moral and physical torture of their wives and by self-torture. They were mostly expressed at late night hours and were connected with a peculiar satisfaction of the "tormenting voluptuousness" (Lemke-Rennert). There was also a sexual excitation with a dissociation between high necessities and dropped possibilities in the sexual sphere against the background of lowered potency and other sexual disorders. Moreover, there was a high level of general excitation with a narrowing of consciousness, vegeto-vascular changes, which are described during coitus, and a satisfaction of sexual necessities by perversions. A visualization of images, related to jealousy was observed, which leads to an increase of the affective shading in delusions. (English abstract was provided as a summary at the beginning of foreign article cited above.) (Author)

271. Ullman, A. D. One against the world. In A. D. Ullman, *To know the difference*. New York: St. Martin's Press, 1960.

One of the many problems of the married male alcoholic is his inability to fulfill his sexual role. Impotence occurs in middle or later stages of his drinking career and is a source of harm to his self-esteem. He tends to lose interest in sex or to act as if his wife had lost interest.

272. Viamontes, J. A. Alcohol abuse and sexual dysfunction. *Medical Aspects of Human Sexuality*, 1974, *8*, 185–186.

In a brief response to a question on chronic alcoholic use and its effect on sexual response, the author states that available studies show without exception a depressant effect on ejaculation and erection. The effect was reported in one study to be temporary although some clinicians observed permanent impairment.

273. Viamontes, J. A. Sexual depressant effect of alcohol. *Medical Aspects of Human Sexuality*, 1975, *9*, 31.

In a question and answer section of this journal, the author is asked to clarify the effect of alcohol on sexual response and to state the degree of permanency of the effect. He responds that alcohol may not abolish sexual motivation but does impair ejaculation, erection, and achievement of orgasm. The effect has been found to be temporary, although there are clinical reports of permanent impairment by the chronic use of alcohol.

274. Vijayasenan, M. E. Alcohol and Sex. *New Zealand Medical Journal*, 1981, *93*, 18–20.

A definite and important association between alcoholism and persistent sexual dysfunction or sexual deviation was determined in the study of 97 male alcoholic inpatients. Pathogenesis and psychogenesis of alcohol-induced sex dysfunction are discussed. (NCALI)

275. Weddige, R. L. Lithium therapy: Episodic drinking and impotence. *Pharmacology, Biochemistry and Behavior*, 1980, *12*, 326.

A 62-year-old man, an episodic drinker diagnosed initially as suffering from bipolar manic-depressive illness, was studied for approximately 7 years. Maintenance therapy with LI2C03 (0.7–0.8 MEQ/liter) failed to modify his drinking behavior, but coadministration of amitriptyline abolished his "craving for alcohol." Impotence occurred during treatment with lithium alone and with combined drug therapy; dynamic psychotherapy and testosterone administration did not alter this. Sexual potency reappeared after cessation of lithium therapy on several occasions. In a 50-year-old patient, sexual impotence also occurred following lithium therapy. (RUCAS)

276. Whalley, L. J. Sexual adjustment of male alcoholics. *Acta Psychiatrica Scandinavica*, 1978, *58*, 281–298.

This study set out to describe the sexual attitudes and behavior of 50 hospitalized alcoholic men by comparing them with a sample of the general population, matched in age and social class. This control sample was identified by random selection from a company register, and subjects were recruited into the study with the assistance of a trade union. All subjects completed the same assessment by semi-structured interview and the Eysenck Inventory of Attitudes to Sex. A method of scoring this questionnaire was derived, and comparison between samples showed the alcoholics differed from the controls only in describing less sexual satisfaction and not in other sexual attitudes. This difference probably arose from the alcoholics' greater interest in sex, loss of erectile potency, and lack of a sexual partner. (Author)

277. Whalley, L. J., & McGuire, R. J. Measuring sexual attitudes. *Acta Psychiatrica Scandinavica*, 1978, *58*, 299–314.

The study set out to examine theoretical and practical aspects of measuring sexual attitudes. Using the replies to a sexual attitude questionnaire developed by Eysenck given to 135 males (50 alcoholics, 50 matched normals, and 35 sex offenders), item and factor analysis led to the composition of 9 short scales measuring sexual satisfaction, heterosexual nervousness, sexual curiosity, tension and hostility, pruriency, sexual repression, heterosexual distaste, and sexual promiscuity. The reliability and validity of the scales are demonstrated and their relationships to each other and to other aspects of sexuality are described. It is pointed out how relevant the scales may be in assessing and monitoring treatment of sexual deviants and others with sex problems. Tentative norms are provided. (Author)

278. Williams, E. Y. The anxiety syndrome in alcoholism. *Psychiatric Quarterly,* 1950, *24,* 782–787.

In the study of 67 alcoholics and a review of 38 cases previously studied, reasons for drinking as given by these patients are listed. It is believed that these reasons reveal symptoms characteristic of the anxiety syndrome. Nervous tension with anxiety appearing at puberty was noted prior to drinking by all patients questioned. Age at onset of drinking tabulated in 67 patients: 4 started before age 11, 5 at 12 and 13, 48 between 14 and 21, 7 at 22 and 24, and 3 over 25. Feelings interpreted as symptoms of anxiety are believed to have served as a basis for drinking in all cases. The symptoms were associated at the outset with sexual frustration; patients drank to "calm the nerves," then needed more alcohol with time; eventually every unpleasant situation called for a drink. Alcohol gave gratification for sexual urges and became a substitute for sexual congress. Increased lack of interest in sex led to divorce. After divorce 30% of patients returned to their parents; another 50% admitted preference for parents rather than spouse. Apparently those who did not get divorced did not do so because their partners were very much in love with them. "In all of the cases where heavy drinking began after puberty, there was an unsatisfactory sexual adjustment or ignorance of sex urges, prior to the drinking habit." Alcoholics drink because of anxiety that starts at puberty. Why others do not resort to alcohol is the question. Literature is reviewed and agreement is expressed with Strecker's idea that the alcoholic is an introvert. Schilder believed that the alcoholic experiences sexual inferiority. (RUCAS)

279. Wyss, R. Alkoholismus und persönlichkeit. [Alcoholism and personality.] *Praxis,* 1970, *59,* 515–518.

The author looks at the causes of alcoholism and contends that only 28% of alcoholic persons show normal sexual behavior. (NCALI)

B. Sex Therapy and Sex Education with Male and Female Alcoholics

280. Barlow, D. H., & Wincze, J. P. Treatment of sexual deviation. In S. R. Leiblum & L. A. Pervin (Eds.), *Principles and practice of sex therapy*. New York: The Guilford Press, 1980.

In discussing contraindications to sex therapy in both homosexual and heterosexual couples, the authors list untreated substance abuse, such as alcoholism, in one or both partners. Two case histories are presented to illustrate the authors' treatment approach. One of these, a case of multiple sexual deviations, involved a 31-year-old man with a history of alcohol abuse. He had begun peeping, exhibiting himself, and indulging in sexual activities with prepubescent girls in his early teens. At 23, he married and temporarily relinquished his old sexual behaviors. Discouraged by his marriage, he began drinking heavily and resuming his exhibitionism and pedophiliac behaviors. Treatment consisted of (a) covert sensitization, focusing on sexual arousal and behavior with prepubescent females, and (b) orgasmic reconditioning to increase the arousal value of adult females. During treatment he was restricted to a hospital ward with no opportunity to drink, and an alcoholism treatment plan was developed to follow the sexual therapy program. However, 6 months after his inpatient course of treatment, he resumed drinking and deviant sexual behavior. The authors conclude that because neither the sex therapy program nor the alcohol treatment program helped him develop adequate coping behaviors and problem-solving skills, stress led to a resumption of drinking, and the deviant sexual behavior followed shortly thereafter.

281. Barnes, J. L., & Schnarch, D. M. A response to "sexual dysfunctions of the alcoholic." *Sexuality and Disability*, 1980, *3*, 291–293.

This article critiques a literature review by Gad-Luther (1980) (see entry 291). The authors question Gad-Luther's conclusions, pointing out problems in generalizing from research conducted with nonalcoholic subjects to alcoholics and failure to differentiate between physiological and subjective components of sexual arousal. Gad-Luther's assertion that sexual dysfunction and alcoholism are pathological entities that share parallel personality dynamics is questioned on the grounds that such an observation is not supported by available research. The authors also take issue with the idea that sexual dysfunction is necessarily pathological. The critique continues by addressing Gad-Luther's pursuit of similarities between sex therapy and alcoholism treatment and

concludes by calling for an integration of the knowledge from the 2 fields.

282. Berenson, D. Sexual counseling with alcoholics. In J. Newman (Ed.), *Sexual counseling for persons with alcoholic problems: Proceedings of a workshop at Pittsburgh, Pennsylvania, January 22–23, 1976*. Pittsburgh, PA: University of Pittsburgh, 1976.

An introduction to sex therapy for couples with alcohol problems is presented using case histories to highlight various methods of treating sexual problems. Sensate focus instruction as a treatment method is discussed, and the importance of obtaining a complete alcohol and sexual history is emphasized. According to the author, sexual counseling is not effective unless the alcohol abuser has ceased drinking for a period of 6 to 18 months.

283. Burger, H., & Rose, N. Sexual impotence. *Medical Journal of Australia*, 1979, *662*, 24–26.

This discussion of types, causes, diagnosis, and management of sexual impotence in men includes a brief section on the cause of impotence in alcoholism. (NCALI)

284. Cerul, M. Basic considerations in sexual counseling. In J. Newman (Ed.), *Sexual counseling for persons with alcohol problems: Proceedings of a workshop at Pittsburgh, Pennsylvania, January 22–23, 1976*. Pittsburgh, PA: University of Pittsburgh, 1976.

A general review of sexual therapies for alcohol abusers is presented. Categories of sexual dysfunction are outlined and problems inherent to each are discussed. Major categories of sexual dysfunction seen in therapy are: (1) impotence, (2) premature ejaculation, (3) retarded ejaculation, (4) female orgasmic dysfunction, and (5) vaginismus. Treatment methods include education, behavior therapy, hypnosis, psychotherapy, and Masters and Johnson-style techniques.

285. Dowsling, J. L. Sex therapy for recovering alcoholics: An essential part of family therapy. *International Journal of the Addictions*, 1980, *15*, 1179–1189.

It is suggested that many recovering alcoholics who complain of sexual dysfunction do not have a clear-cut organic basis for their problem. Sexual recovery is essential though, because alcoholism and sexual problems have had a detrimental effect on family life, and family support is important to recovery. It is suggested that sex should be viewed as another aspect of communication which may need attention. Sex therapy for recovering alcoholics is seen as an opportunity to begin building self-esteem, a unifying force for the couple, and as a reinforcement for sobriety. (NCALI)

286. Ferrant, J. P., Benard, J. Y., & Laudier, J. Une infinie tendresse. [Infinite tenderness.] *Revue de l'Alcoolisme,* 1979, *25,* 161–164.

The restoration of a couple's sex life, after it has been disrupted by conflicts due to alcohol misuse by one of the partners, is discussed in terms of the demands this task makes upon the physician after the patient has regained self-control and sobriety. Although sexology courses have been part of the medical school curriculum for some time, many physicians are still unprepared to handle these problems. The effects of alcoholism on a couple's life are comparable with major bone fractures and severe diseases in that, after physical healing, only a thorough re-education of the patient in the use of the affected limb or faculty makes total functional restoration possible. The physician should try to induce both partners to practice tolerance and forgiveness for the partner's shortcomings and recognize one's own, to give priority to the partner's pleasure, and to develop regard and empathy for the partner's feelings, needs, and longings. (RUCAS)

287. Finkle, A. L. Sexual impotency: Current knowledge and treatment: I. Urology/sexuality clinic. *Urology,* 1980, *16,* 442–452.

In a discussion of etiology and treatment of sexual impotence in men it is noted that the effect of alcohol on the mechanisms of potency is not fully understood. It is thought that both organic and psychological components are involved. (RUCAS)

288. Fleetwood, M. A. *Significant issues cited by five women in recovery from alcoholism: The first and second years.* Paper presented at the Mount Holyoke Conference on Women and Alcohol, South Hadley, MA, March 1980.

Five women in recovery from alcoholism were interviewed in 2-hour sessions. The respondents were (1) a 19-year-old woman with a history of family violence and street experience; (2) a 42-year-old divorced parent; (3) a 50-year-old suburban housewife and mother of 2 adopted children; (4) a 37-year-old career woman and self-identified lesbian; and (5) a 27-year-old Black woman, head of a household with 3 children. Only the Black woman had 2 years of continuous sobriety at the time of the interview; the other women were in their first year of sobriety. A questionnaire containing questions pertaining to self-concept, personal identity, medical history, relationships with others, work, sexuality, and spirituality was used in taping the interviews. Significant issues or common experiences cited by the 5 women in early sobriety are listed. Suggestions are offered for improving the treatment of women recovering from alcoholism. A copy of the questionnaire used in the interviews is provided. (NCALI)

289. Fleit, L. *Alcohol and sexuality: A handbook for the counselor/therapist.* Arlington, VA: H/P Publishing Co., 1970.

This handbook intended for sex therapists includes a brief chapter on sexual functioning during and after recovery from alcoholism. (RUCAS)

290. Franek, B., & Franek, M. *Sexual rehabilitation in alcoholism recovery.* Paper presented at the Twenty-seventh International Institute on the Prevention and Treatment of Alcoholism, Vienna, June 1981.

In this paper, the authors describe some case studies of persons with chronic alcoholism and coexisting psychosexual disturbances, and discuss sexual rehabilitation in alcoholism recovery. It is recommended that every sex therapist become thoroughly familiar with the symptomatology of early and intermediate alcoholism. (NCALI)

291. Gad-Luther, I. Sexual dysfunctions of the alcoholic. *Sexuality and Disability,* 1980, *3,* 273–290.

After reviewing the theories proposed as models for alcoholism, a picture seems to emerge that may serve to incorporate the sexual dysfunctions occurring in chronic alcoholism. So far, neither the clinical anecdotal data nor the recent research on nonalcoholics conducted in controlled laboratory conditions could explain the persistence of sexual dysfunctions after years of sobriety. The seemingly paradoxical appearance, during periods of alcohol abstinence, of a more severe symptom of sexual malfunction—the total lack of sexual desire—may be conceived as an attempt to compensate a psychodynamic imbalance: as alcoholism is alleviated, the sexual dysfunction is aggravated. Therefore, in order to be effective, sex therapy for the alcoholic has to address itself at the same time to the intrapersonal dynamics, to the interpersonal system, as well as to the actual presenting sexual complaints. (Author)

292. Gad-Luther, I., & Dailey, J. Understanding sex and alcohol. *Sexology,* 1979, *45,* 38–41.

There are no aftercare programs concerned with the sexual malfunctions common in alcoholics. It is suggested that the field of sex therapy can make a positive contribution in this area. (RUCAS)

293. Gad-Luther, I., & Dickman, D. Psychosexual therapy with recovering alcoholics: a pilot study. *Journal of Sex Education and Therapy,* 1979, *1,* 11–16.

Five recovered alcoholics and their spouses were given the LoPiccolo Sexual Interaction Inventory (SII), the Locke-Wallace Marital Adjustment Test, and the Berger Self-Acceptance/Other Acceptance Test before and after 10 3-hour sessions of psychosexual multiple team therapy. The results indicated significant (p–.05) changes in the total adjustment, mate acceptance (male of female), perceptual accuracy (female of male), and self-acceptance (female) scales of the SII; impressive (p–.01) changes of the male Self-Acceptance on the Berger test; and a trend (p–.10) toward improvement of the female Marital Adjustment on the Locke-Wallace test.

These results seem to support the hypotheses that a multi-dimensional therapy such as the new sexual therapy is an appropriate approach to a psychophysiological problem such as alcoholism. In view of these results it is believed that a further study of the effect of psychosexual therapy on recovered alcoholics on a greater number of subjects is warranted. (Author)

294. Gallavardin, J. P. *Homoopathische beeinflussung von charakter, trunksucht und sexualtrieb. [Homeopathic effect on character, alcoholism and sex drive.]* Heidelberg: Karl F. Haug Verlag, 1978.

This book contains German translations of writings by Gallavardin, including an article published in French in 1889, with reports of cases of alcohol intoxication and alcoholism successfully treated according to the principles of homeopathy. It is claimed that half of the alcoholics seen could be cured in this way, as long as their condition was not hereditary. A list of 14 primary substances (e.g., sulfur, opium, petroleum, mercury, arsenic, calcium or magnesium carbonate, staphisagria) is presented, one of which is to be added surreptitiously to the alcoholic's food. It is stressed that the substance should be chosen on the basis of the alcoholic's psychological and physical characteristics and symptoms, and indications for each of the substances are presented in detail. In all, over 40 stubstances have been recommended for treating alcoholism and aberrant behavior associated with drunkenness. (RUCAS)

295. Gerevich, J. A Moravcsik Klub müködése. [The activity of the Moravcsik Club.] *Alkohológia,* 1979, *10,* 73–76.

The "Moravcsik" psychohygienic club of treated alcoholics was founded in February 1977 as a part of the University Psychiatric Clinic's day hospital in Budapest. The membership is open and consists of 26 former alcoholics, 8 supporting members, and 12 former mental patients. Four members relapsed during the first and one during the second year of the club's existence. The club shares its therapists and many of its programs and activities (trips, games, exhibitions) with the day hospital and receives help from the district alcoholism service and various other organizations. The activities include among others a "disco" club, a cinema club (which included showings of 'sex-centered" short films to stimulate the sexually inactive patients) and organization of and attendance at exhibitions. (RUCAS)

296. Hawkins, R. O. *Sex education for alcohol counselors.* Paper presented at Eleventh National Sex Institute of the American Association of Sex Educators, Counselors, and Therapists, Washington, DC, March 1978.

This paper discusses the need for sex education for alcoholism counselors and describes 2 programs, a single 2-hour lecture and discussion and a 10-session, 20-hour workshop designed to fill the need. The author observes: (a) a deficit in factual information on sexuality in general, (b) a lack in awareness of alcoholics' sexual concerns, and (c) the need for professionals to explore their own attitudes. The need for counselors to develop a nonjudgmental attitude and to increase self-awareness of their attitudes is stressed since the counselor's attitudes may be a barrier to approaching the client's sexual problems or may interfere with the counselor's providing adequate help. In addition to sexual dysfunction problems, the client may need to address issues around homosexuality or incest.

297. Hoon, E. F., Murphy, W. D., Coleman, E., & Scott, C. *Sexual enhancement for female alcoholics.* Paper presented at the Fourth Annual Southeastern Regional Conference of the American Association of Sex Educators, Counselors and Therapists, Charleston, SC, October 1979.

A sexual enhancement program for inpatient alcoholic females was designed and implemented. Some encouraging preliminary outcome data were obtained. A closed group format was chosen to create and maintain a sufficient level of trust that would free group members to share feelings and past experiences openly. Participation was voluntary. To avoid random attendance, patients who missed 2 sessions were dropped. There were 2 sets of group leaders: female co-leaders, or a male and female co-leader team. Their role was to introduce specific exercises and topics, to serve as timekeepers, and generally to facilitate the group. Initial group sessions were quite structured, with later sessions gradually becoming less structured and more personal. The outline of the group could be divided into 4 stages: sex education, sexual awareness, sexual dysfunction, and sexual assertiveness. Pre- and postgroup measures were taken on communications effectiveness, marital happiness, sexual knowledge, sexual attitudes, and sexual functioning. The group experience increased information about sex, marital happiness, comfort in talking about sex, and sexual arousability.

298. Howard, D., & Howard, N. *Touching me, touching you.* Columbia, MO: Family Training Center, 1977.

This is a sexual enhancement manual intended for use by the patient to assist his or her initial self-assessment of sexual feelings, needs, desires, and fantasies. The authors share their personal experiences with developing their sexuality, including the male author's bout with alcoholism. Use of alcohol can interfere with the development of appropriate and adequate interpersonal skills which, in turn, disrupts or prevents intimate relationships. Patterns involving anxiety and concern for performance develop and are complicated by the detrimental physiological effects of alcohol on performance. The female alcoholic drinks to feel feminine and sexy, yet it is a futile attempt since she does not know what feminine is. Both male and female alcoholics could benefit from general sex education.

299. Kaplan, H. S. *The new sex therapy.* New York: Brunner/Mazel, 1974, 86–89; 98; 445; 463–465.

The adverse effect of alcohol on sexual functioning is discussed. Excessive alcohol use and alcoholism make for a poor prognosis in sex therapy. Severe, active alcoholics are considered inappropriate candidates for sex therapy.

300. Kaplan, H. S. *Disorders of sexual desire and other new concepts and techniques in sex therapy.* New York: Simon & Schuster, 1979, 81; 127–129; 203; 211.

Some drugs, such as alcohol, depress sexual desire. Drug and alcohol abusers have a poor prognosis for sex therapy and should not be accepted for treatment until the habit is under control. A table presents commonly used drugs, their mechanisms of action, and their effects on the phases of sexual response. In one of the case histories illustrating the inhibiting influence of anger on sexual desire, the wife's anger over discovering her husband's past history of alcohol abuse figured in the etiology of the couple's sexual problems.

301. Kern, J. C., & Hawkins, R. O. Integrating education on sexuality into an alcoholism treatment program. *Journal of Psychiatric Treatment and Evaluation,* 1980, *2,* 37–43.

This article describes the activities involved in integrating information and counseling on sexuality into an existing alcoholism program. The needs of alcoholics and their families for counseling around sexuality in the early stages of sobriety has been well-documented. However, staff of alcoholism agencies are reluctant to acknowledge the needs of clients in this area. This paper describes a series of training sessions for staff extending over a 3-year period. The training helped them clarify their own values regarding sexuality, and provided workshop experience for designing educational material for clients. Guidelines are provided regarding the method of implementation of staff training, selection of staff to be "experts" in human sexuality, and related issues. (Author)

302. Lavengood, R. W. Nonsurgical treatment of impotence. *Annals of Plastic Surgery,* 1978, *1,* 239–240.

Various nonpsychological causes of impotence are pointed out, and it is suggested that alcohol consumption should always be questioned in such cases.

303. Lemere, F. Sexual impairement in recovered alcoholics. *Medical Aspects of Human Sexuality,* 1976, *10,* 69–70.

Sexual dysfunction occurring during active drinking may persist after the alcoholic has achieved sobriety. This may be caused by a resurgence of psychosexual inhibitions that had been suppressed by alcohol or by physiological damage done by alcohol. Impotence may be reversed in a few months, and most patients are best left to work out their temporary impotence in their own way. Reassurance and perhaps Vitamin E or small doses of testosterone (for their placebo effect) may be helpful. Should impotence continue beyond several months, marital counseling may be called for. A penile prosthesis may be considered should the impotence prove permanent.

304. Lobitz, W. C., & Lobitz, G. K. Clinical assessment in the treatment of sexual dysfunctions. In J. LoPiccolo & L. LoPiccolo (Eds.), *Handbook of sex therapy.* New York: Plenum Press, 1978.

Because of the adverse effects of alcohol on sexual response, alcoholics frequently develop erectile dysfunctions. Although performance anxiety may have developed in response to initial episodes of erectile dysfunction due to alcohol, patients rarely associated their sexual problem with their drinking. Sex therapy is contraindicated for alcoholics unless they have been able to control their drinking for at least 6 months. (Author)

305. Malloy, E. S. Strategies in sexual counseling in alcoholic marriages. In J. Newman (Ed.), *Sexual counseling for persons with alcohol problems: Proceedings of a workshop at Pittsburgh, Pennsylvania, January 22–23, 1976.* Pittsburgh, PA: University of Pittsburgh, 1976.

Sexual counseling in alcoholic marriages is discussed, particularly the decision as to when or if it is appropriate. Sexual dysfunction as an inevitable side effect of alcohol abuse is also examined. Ongoing alcoholism is seen as one factor mitigating against the success of brief-treatment sexual therapy. It is stressed that resolution of relationship difficulties in the alcoholic marriage is necessary before sexual problems can be discussed rationally. The difficulties of sexual relationships are likely to be exacerbated by alcoholism.

306. Masters, W. H., & Johnson, V. E. *Human sexual inadequacy.* Boston: Little, Brown, 1970, 160; 163–169; 183–185.

Alcoholism or a specific incident of excessive alcohol intake is the second most common cause of secondary impotence. A case history is presented, illustrating the onset and course through therapy of secondary impotence induced by a specific incident of alcohol–induced erectile failure.

307. Miller, P. M., & Mastria, M. A. Sex counseling. In P. M. Miller & M. A. Mastria, *Alternatives to alcohol abuse: A social learning model.* Champaign, IL: Research Press, 1977.

Alcoholic men and women often suffer some form of sexual problem. Promiscuity may occur more readily; inability to perform may result from the physiologically depressing effects of alcohol; the interpersonal relationship upon which a satisfying sexual relationship is based may be distorted because of the personal problems of the alcoholics. The counselor should be sensitive and well-informed about sexual anatomy and counseling techniques and should function as a role model with open, responsible attitudes toward sex. Assessment, diagnosis, and counselling techniques based on the behavior therapy literature are discussed in detail.

308. Milner, G. *Drug awareness: Drugs and drink—awareness and action.* Melbourne, Australia: Perfect Publishing Co., 1979.

This handbook on legal and illegal drugs includes information on alcohol, including lethal dose, metabolism, related problems, and beverage strengths and quantities in a general framework of topics intended to help parents, teachers, service club members, journalists, therapists, and other professionals who deal with drug misuse. Topics include social, legal, and general treatment and rehabilitation considerations. Methodologies such as social skills and relaxation training, sex, behavior and family therapy, transactional analysis, Alcoholics Anonymous, and therapeutic communities are discussed. (RUCAS)

309. Mudd, J. W. Physical examination in marital and sexual disorders. In D. W. Abse, E. M. Nash, & L. M. R. Louden (Eds.), *Marital & sexual counseling in medical practice* (2nd ed.). New York: Harper & Row, 1974.

Marital or sexual disturbance may be the first indication of organic disease. Mild psychological problems may be due to organic disease and have deleterious social consequences for the patient. Organic causes should be ruled out before assuming that dysfunction is psychogenic. Overindulgence in alcohol is among the conditions that may produce mild personality disturbances. Severe alcoholism may be either cause or effect in a man's loss of libido. Atrophic tests may indicate severe alcoholism. Physical examinations by the patient's physician-counselor are contraindicated for individuals with severe psychopathology and for patients who are involved in long-term, psychoanalytically oriented treatment. In these cases, examination referral may be indicated.

310. Newman, J. (Ed.). *Sexual counseling for persons with alcohol problems: Proceedings of a workshop at Pittsburgh, Pennsylvania, January 22–23, 1976.* Pittsburgh, PA: University of Pittsburgh, 1976.

This book contains transcripts of the presentations and discussions on sexual difficulties frequently encountered in working with people with alcohol problems. Clinical data and thinking about sex therapy are presented for alcoholism counselors to consider.

311. Page, A. Counselling. In Camberwell Council on Alcoholism, *Women and alcohol.* New York: Tavistock Publications, 1980.

The most common types of psychological treatment for alcoholism in women, including individual counselling, group therapy, and marriage therapy, are described. In addition, it is suggested that sex therapy may also have a place in the treatment of women drinkers, because of the frequent sexual difficulties experienced by them and their partners. An alcoholic woman may benefit from a combination of counselling approaches, each having a specific purpose. She may then join a support group, practice new social skills, and find resources other than a professional counselor to help her toward Alcoholics Anonymous, new friendships, or women's groups.

312. Redmond, A. C., & Whitfield, C. L. Alcohol and sexuality. In C. L. Whitfield (Ed.), *The patient with alcoholism & other drug problems: A clinical approach for physicians & helping professionals.* Chicago: Yearbook Medical Publication, 1981.

This chapter was written for medical professionals who are called upon to assist patients with alcohol and sexual problems. To prepare the reader, the authors begin by describing sexual development throughout the normal life cycle from conception to adulthood. They then explore major discrepancies between social beliefs about the effect of alcohol on sexuality and recent scientific data demonstrating the physiological effects of alcohol use on the sexual response cycle, i.e., the belief that alcohol enhances sexual responding versus laboratory demonstrations that alcohol interferes with erectile and ejaculatory responding. Various etiological factors that lead to sexual dysfunction in the alcoholic are discussed along with changes in sexual functioning that accompany the progress of alcoholism and recovery during sobriety. The authors recommend that sex education and counselling be included in alcoholism treatment and make suggestions for referring a recovering alcoholic to a specialist for sex therapy. They also suggest that a competent therapist explore his/her own feelings and attitudes about sexuality since the therapist's comfort with the topic determines the client's ability to discuss sexual difficulties.

313. Santa Clara County Alcoholism Program. *Alcoholism and sexuality workshop.* Unpublished report, 1976. (Available from Park Alameda Health Facility, 976 Lenzen Avenue, San Jose, CA 95126.)

This is a report on the workshop series. The workshop was of educational intent, providing a forum for exploration of sexual problems among alcoholics. Workshop leaders emphasized the importance of openness and self-awareness, as well as the need for accurate information, with regard to sexuality.

314. Semmens, J. P., & Semmens, F. J. Premature ejaculation and impotence: Male problems with gynecologic implications. *Clinical Obstetrics and Gynecology,* 1978, *21,* 223–233.

Inquiry into sex therapy for male sexual dysfunction occurs more frequently in the gynecologist's office than in that of any other medical specialist. The existence of a sexual problem in the male partner should be suspected as a contributing factor in primary or secondary female nonorgasmic response. The existence of sexual problems may surface only after recurrent office visits for minor gynecological complaints. Premature ejaculation and impotence, the most commonly presented forms of male sexual dysfunction, are described, and etiology and treatment are discussed. Alcoholism figures as a major cause of impotence through its effect on physiological and endocrine functions, as well as through the psychological satiation derived from drinking rather than from contact with a sexual partner.

315. Stump, C. C. *Alcoholism and sexuality: A sexual awareness program for alcoholism treatment facilities.* Paper presented at the National Council on Alcoholism Forum, New Orleans, April 1981.

A simple program of sexual awareness for the alcoholic patient and his/her partner is presented. The program is designed as a guide for the professional alcoholism counsellor. Six major areas of sexual awareness are introduced and discussed. The importance of assessing each patient for potential sexual dysfunction problems is stressed. Guidelines are presented for identifying and treating these problems or for referring such patients to other sources for help. In addition to the program, counsellors must have an understanding of their own sexuality and their personal values system. Alcoholism is considered to be the primary problem and must be dealt with before any other type of therapy can be attempted. (NCALI)

316. Van Thiel, D. H., & Lester, R. Therapy of sexual dysfunction in alcohol abusers: A pandora's box. *Gastroenterology*, 1977, *72*, 1354–1356.

The introduction of therapeutic intervention in the sexual dysfunction associated with alcoholism and/or liver disease presents a complex problem. No one form of treatment appears to be free from problems. Administration of testosterone might increase beard growth and restore potency but would have no effect on inadequate spermatogenesis or would further impair it, and would have no effect on signs of hyperestrogenization. An already suppressed hypothalamus-pituitary function would be further inhibited, thereby diminishing the gonadotropin stimulus for deficient gonads. Treatment with gonadotropins would be financially and technically impractical. Clomiphene has been reported to produce dramatic, albeit transient, effects by interrupting the steroid feedback control of the hypothalamus resulting in increases in plasma gonadotropin concentrations. Problems arise when considering complication from long-term administration. Because clomiphene is a weakly estrogenic agent, there may be undesirable effects on patients who show signs of hyperestrogenization. Also, little is known about effects of prolonged use on gonad and liver electrolyte and fluid balances or on portal hypertension. Some patients are unresponsive to clomiphene; the therapeutic effect is restricted to certain symptoms. Finally, one cannot be certain of the permanence of favorable results, especially in the face of continued ethanol ingestion.

317. Whitfield, C. L. *Alcohol and sexual function* (Report based on paper presented at a seminar sponsored by the Council on Alcoholism for Fairfax and Springfield, Virginia, 1978). Baltimore, MD: Essex Bookshop, 1978.

The effects of chronic alcohol consumption on sexual function and behavior are discussed in terms of: (1) factors (historical and current) implicated in the etiology of sexual dysfunction, (2) alcohol toxicity, and (3) the inability of alcoholic patients to form intimate relationships. These factors, it is stated, should be taken into consideration in counselling any alcoholic patient. An approach to managing alcohol problems is illustrated by means of a diagnostic and therapeutic flow chart for sexual dysfunction and alcohol use. (NCALI)

318. Whitley, M. J. Sexuality and substance abuse: Treatment for the troubled family. (Training module 8—summary.) In D. J. Ottenberg & E. E. Madden (Eds.), *Proceedings of the 13th Annual Eagleville Conference. Substance Abuse: The Family in Trouble, May 1980*. Eagleville, PA: Eagleville Hospital and Rehabilitation Center, 1980.

A brief summary of a training module on sexuality and substance abuse treatment for the troubled family is presented. (NCALI)

319. Zizic, V., Fridman, V., & Despotovic. A. Mogucnost lecenja impotencije alkoholicara. [Possibilities for the treatment of impotency in alcoholics.] *Anali Klinicke Bolnice*, 1967, *6*, 221–230.

The frequency of sexual impotence in alcoholics was found to be unexpectedly small (3.9%). On this basis and in view of the long period of prior addiction, it is concluded that the action of alcohol as an exogenous toxin on the development of sexual impotence is negligible. The possibility of the development of sexual impotence being due to the use of disulfiram is discarded. The methods for the treatment of sexual impotence in alcoholics, as well as some theoretical and personal views drawn from 33 cases observed and treated over a long period, are presented. (English abstract and English title were provided as a summary at the end of foreign article cited above.) (Author)

III. Social Problems and Cultural Issues Relating to Alcohol and Sexuality

Introduction
A. Sexual Deviance and Crime
   1. Rape
   2. Incest
   3. Child Molesting
   4. Miscellaneous
B. Venereal Disease
C. Alcoholism and Homosexuality
   1. Both Sexes (or Gender Unspecified)
   2. Females
   3. Males
D. Cross-Cultural and Historical Reports
E. Alcohol and Sexuality in the Media

Introduction

The sections in this chapter contain explorations into the relationship between sex and alcohol as reflected in history, culture, and social problems. The first section examines the role of alcoholism and alcohol use in sexual deviance and sex crimes. The reader will find survey reports on the rate of alcoholism among incarcerated prisoners and on the frequency with which sex offenders report alcohol involvement in their crimes. Information on the victim's involvement with alcohol is also found in this chapter. Studies of clinical records of sex offenders and deviants and case histories provide psychological insights into the relationship between alcohol, sexual crimes, and sexual deviance. The studies and commentary presented here come from throughout the world and represent various points in history. Section A, which treats reports on sexual deviance and crime, is subdivided into those dealing with rape, incest, or child molestation. Publications that cover more than one of these crimes or other types of sex deviation/crime relationships have been placed in the group labeled "Miscellaneous." The miscellaneous group also contains reports on unusual forms of deviance, such as autocastration and satyriasis, and material on prostitution.

Section B of this chapter compiles research reports on the role of alcohol use and abuse in relation to venereal disease. These papers address how alcohol use affects the circumstances under which venereal disease is contracted, failure to comply with treatment programs, severity of symptoms, and reinfection.

The materials in Section C deal with alcoholism among homosexuals. The prevalence of alcoholism among homosexuals and the inadequacies of existing alcoholism treatment services in addressing the special needs of sexual minorities are primary topics of many articles. Some writers provide guidelines for improving services and developing outreach programs that are appropriate for gays and lesbians. Others provide information about the development of alcoholism within the homosexual subculture. Published resource guides listing alcoholism treatment services for gays are included in this chapter. Within this chapter, articles are grouped by gender of subject with entries addressing both lesbians and gay men placed first, followed by articles on female homosexuals exclusively, and concluding with articles on males. The reader who is interested in psychoanalytic propositions causally linking alcoholism with latent or overt homosexuality is referred to Chapter IV, Section B, Psychoanalytic Commentary.

Section D cites anthropological studies and historical reports on the cultural meaning of drinking practices as they relate to sexual customs. These are the result of examinations of historical records, observations and interviews in the field, and analyses of folktales. The cross-cultural studies are predominantly of societies in the Western Hemisphere: natives of North America, Central American villagers, American Indian societies, present-day ethnic groups, and modern urban Indians. However, some information is available on cultures in other parts of the world as well. Historical studies, too, describe customs linking sexual behavior and drinking practices. The reports touch diverse places and times, such as ancient China, seventeenth century England, and the American Old West. Historical information which primarily focuses on alcohol as an aphrodisiac is contained in the "Alcohol as an Aphrodisiac" section of Chapter I.

Section E, the concluding section in this chapter, provides a look at the relationship between sex and alcohol as represented in the media. The citations here are mostly studies of advertising practices making use of sex to market alcohol.

A. Sexual Deviance and Crime

1. Rape

320. Amir, M. Alcohol and forcible rape. *British Journal of Addiction*, 1967, *62*, 219–232.

Of the 646 cases of forcible rape investigated by the Philadelphia Police Department in 1958 and 1960, alcohol played a role (victim or offender had been drinking) in 217 cases: in 10% of victims only, in 3% of offenders only, and in 21% of both victim and offender. Alcohol was present in the victim, offender, or both, in 42% of the 44 cases in which a White man was involved, in 24% of the 173 cases in which a Black man was involved, in 26% of the 16 cases in which a White woman was victimized, and in 20% of the 201 cases in which a Black woman was the victim. Women who were drunk or drinking in a public place with strangers were more vulnerable to rape by their drinking companions. The lone Black woman was most victimized. In all cases where alcohol was a factor in the offender only, force was used upon the victim; a significant relation was found between alcohol in the offender only and infliction of a brutal beating on the victim. The drinking Black offender was most often involved in violence. Sexual humiliation occurred in 44% of the cases where alcohol was a factor. There was a significant association between weekend consumption of alcohol and the high proportion of forcible rapes on weekends. (RUCAS)

321. Enos, W. F., & Beyer, J. C. Prostatic acid phosphatase, aspermia, and alcoholism in rape cases. *Journal of Forensic Science*, 1980, *25*, 353–356.

In 2 rape cases, oral, vaginal, or rectal smears of the victims were negative for spermatozoa; presence of prostatic acid phosphatase was the only laboratory evidence that vaginal penetration and ejaculation had taken place. Both attackers were long-term alcoholics who had children, which supports the fact that alcoholism with or without cirrhosis is one of the most frequent etiological factors in aspermia. (RUCAS)

322. Gagnon, J. H. *Human sexualities*. Oakland, NJ: Scott, Foresman and Company, 1977, 310–311.

Imprisoned rapists may not be representative of all rapists. With a moderate amount of social skill, a man may rape many times without being arrested or convicted of the crime. Imprisoned rapists are in many ways socially incompetent. Their conduct may be characterized by violence, poor judgment that has been further deteriorated by alcohol intoxication or explosive and unpredictable behavior. For these men, sexual behavior can be placed in the context of other behavior: general aggressiveness, heedless lifestyle, the confusions of alcohol, and problems with sexual repression.

323. Gerson, L. W., & Preston, D. A. Alcohol consumption and the incidence of violent crime. *Journal of Studies on Alcohol*, 1979, *40*, 307–312.

Multiple regression was used to examine the effect of alcohol consumption on rates of violent crime (e.g., homicide, assault, rape, sexual assault, and threatening behavior) in an urban, industrialized region of Canada. Information on violent crimes was obtained from the regional police who, for this study, coded crimes as alcohol- or nonalcohol-related. Criteria for being coded alcohol-related were: there was a violation of a specific statute regulating use of alcohol, the victim had been drinking or was intoxicated, the event occurred in or in connection with a licensed establishment, or alcohol was mentioned in the description of the incident. Alcohol consumption was based on sales reports from the Liquor Control Board of Ontario and Brewer's Warehousing. Demographic data were obtained from the regional planning department, census data, and tax enumeration. Mean family income and alcohol consumption accounted for 83.9% of the variation in crime rates; income alone related to the largest proportion, 67.9%. Alcohol consumption in licensed establishments was highly associated with rate of violent crime in that area. Alcohol was involved in 60% of the rapes; 19.1% of the indecent assaults; 49.1% of marital assaults.

324. Groth, A. N., & Burgess, W. Male rape: Offenders and victims. *American Journal of Psychiatry*, 1980, *137*, 806–810.

Male rape in a community setting was investigated in 22 cases. The offender gained sexual control of the victim by entrapment, i.e., getting him drunk (3 cases), by intimidation, or by physical force. For all offenders the sexual assault was an act of retaliation, an expression of power, and an assertion of strength and manhood. The impact of rape on the male victims was similar to that on female victims. (RUCAS)

325. Johnson, S. D., Gibson, L., & Linden, R. Alcohol and rape in Winnipeg, 1966–1975. *Journal of Studies on Alcohol*, 1978, *39*, 1887–1894.

The role of alcohol in 217 rapes reported to the Winnipeg City Police Department during the 10-year period 1966–1975 was examined. Alcohol was present in 72.4% of the rapes, both parties had been drinking in 38.7% of all cases, the rapist only in 24.4%, and the victim only in 9.2%. Alcohol increased the likelihood of force being used, the relationship being weakest when alcohol had been used by the victim alone (gamma = .18) and strongest when both rapist and victim had been drinking (gamma = .35). Of the 191 cases in which data on injury were available, 113 resulted in injury to the victim, the likelihood of injury to the victim being greatest if she alone had been drinking (gamma = .65), weakest if only the offender had been drinking (gamma = .06), and intermediate if both parties had been drinking (gamma = .26). While drinking rapists were involved in 63.1% of all the 217 cases, they committed only 59.5% of the 74 rapes involving especially vulnerable victims (mentally or physically handicapped, very young or very old, working late, living alone, unclothed or sleeping at the time of the rape, intoxicated). However, they were more likely than nondrinking offenders to rape handicapped or intoxicated women. The data provide evidence that the situation of drinking may facilitate rape; 83% of the rapes classified as spontaneous involved alcohol, while 55% of those characterized as "planned" were preceded by drinking. Some of the findings are compared with similar data on rapes reported in Philadelphia and Toronto. (RUCAS)

326. Kaufman, A., Divasto, P., Jackson, R., Voorhees, D., & Christy, J. Male rape victims: Noninstitutionalized assault. *American Journal of Psychiatry*, 1980, *137*, 221–223.

Fourteen male rape victims treated in a county hospital emergency room over a 39-month period were compared with 100 randomly selected female rape victims treated over the same period. The attacker had been drinking in 2 of the 3 cases of homosexual rape described in detail. (RUCAS)

327. Peters, J. J. Commentary on alcohol and rape. *Medical Aspects of Human Sexuality*, 1975, *9*, 65.

Among sex offenders treated in small, psychoanalytic groups at Philadelphia General Hospital's Center for Studies in Sexual Deviance, 50% of the pedophiles (i.e., offenders who attempted intercourse with females age 12 years or less) committed the offense under the influence of excessive alcohol. The dynamics usually included rejection by the adult female partner, increased alcohol consumption, and seduction of the child who was generally known to the offender. Therapeutic goals focus upon control of alcohol consumption.

328. Rabkin, J. G. The epidemiology of forcible rape. *American Journal of Orthopsychiatry*, 1979, *49*, 634–647.

Problems of measurement of the incidence of rape are considered, and empirical findings are summarized regarding prevalence, demographic and psychiatric characteristics of offenders, spatial and temporal distribution of offenses, victim-offender relationships, and evidence about recidivism and progression of crimes. Findings are discussed in the framework of blame models and their implications for treatment and prevention. The role of alcohol is briefly discussed. (Author)

329. Rada, R. T. *Alcoholism and forcible rape.* Paper presented at the meeting of the American Psychological Association, Detroit, May 1974.

The author collected data from 77 subjects who were patients of Atascadero State Hospital, committed for forcible rape,

and concluded that 50% of the rapists had been drinking at the time of assault. Forty-three percent had been drinking heavily, and 35% were diagnosed as alcoholic. In comparison to nonalcoholic rapists, alcoholic rapists were more likely to be drinking at the time of the rape, were more likely to have a history of prior use of drugs other than alcohol, and were more likely to have been using drugs in conjunction with alcohol at the time of the rape. The author calls for cooperation between treatment programs for sex offenders and treatment programs for alcoholic people, and for more follow-up treatment.

330. Rada, R. T. Alcohol and rape. *Medical Aspects of Human Sexuality*, 1975, *9*, 48–65.

Recent data and theoretical material on the relationships between alcohol, alcoholism, and the commission of violent sexual crimes are reported, and several case histories are presented as examples. An attempt is made to differentiate between 3 alcohol/rape situations: rape involving an alcoholic offender, rape involving a drinking offender, and rape that may be triggered or catalyzed by alcohol. It is believed that the rapist seems more concerned about control and power in the rape situation than with sex itself. The need for further research relating to the effect of alcohol on male plasma testosterone is stressed.

331. Rada, R. T. Alcoholism and forcible rape. *American Journal of Psychiatry*, 1975, *132*, 444–446.

Data collected from detailed autobiographies of 77 convicted rapists revealed that 50% of them were drinking at the time of the rape and that 35% were alcoholics. This strong association between alcoholism and forcible rape highlights the importance of follow-up treatment programs for the alcoholic sex offender; such programs should focus on adequate control of his drinking behavior as well as on his sexual adjustment. (Author)

332. Schuster, R. Beteiligung von frauen an alkoholdelikten in Mittelhessen von 1952 bis 1974. [The share of women in alcohol-related offenses in central Hesse from 1952 to 1974.] *Beitrage zur Gerichtlichen Medizin*, 1979, *37*, 207–212.

The involvement of women in alcohol-related offenses in central Hesse, Federal Republic of Germany, was studied by analyzing the blood alcohol archives for 1952–1974. The proportion of women grew from 1% (8 of 721 persons) in 1952 to 3% (14 of 450) in 1974 and an estimated 5% in 1975. Of 987 women tested during that period, 686 were involved in traffic offenses and 287 in criminal offenses. No significant correlation could be found between age and offense category (traffic vs. criminal offenses), though the modal age was somewhat lower for traffic than for criminal offenders (20–24 vs. 24–29 years). The modal blood alcohol concentrations (BAC) were 0.11–0.20% in traffic offenses and 0.16–0.25% in criminal offenses. Seventeen women committed homicide, 74 crimes against property, 48 assault, and 60 were victims of rape. The BAC tests were negative in 132 of the 987 women. (RUCAS)

333. Smith, J. W. Commentary on alcohol and rape. *Medical Aspects of Human Sexuality,* 1975, *9,* 60–62; 65.

Alcohol and rape can be regarded as a facet of alcohol and violence in general. As with other forms of personal violence, alcohol is involved in about 50% of the cases, based on verbal and written reports of offenders and witnesses. Alcohol contributes to violent crime in its use by the victim, reducing the victim's ability to disengage or defend herself. Estimates of the rate in which alcohol is found in the victim are 20–30%. The persons most likely to commit rape are those with a sociopathic personality. Persons who are likely to commit rape and other types of assaultive behavior are also likely to drink. However, it is not correct to say that those who are alcoholics are, because of their alcoholism, more likely to commit rape.

334. Tóth, T. Az alkoholizmus szociálpolitikai, kriminológiai és viktimológiai jellemzöi, II. rész. [The sociopolitical, criminological and victimological characteristics of alcoholism. Part II.] *Alkohológia,* 1979, *10,* 77–83.

Various statistics on alcohol involvement among victims of criminal offenses in Hungary are presented, and reasons for the high rate of crimes against people under the influence of alcohol and alcoholics are discussed. The national statistics for 1976 show that persons under the influence of alcohol perpetrated 26.3% and were the victims of 5.6% of all criminal offenses against person and property; they constituted 25.7% of the offenders and 25.3% of the victims of murder, 0% and 44.4% of offenders and victims, respectively, of manslaughter, 17.0% and 20.3% of minor and 14.7% and 16.8% of severe bodily injury, 46.7% and 0% of attacks against police, 34.6% and 22.3% of disorderly conduct, 10.7% and 5.6% of sexual coercion, 14.1% and 41.0% of fraud. In 1968–1974, in 21%, 26%, and 21% of murders, both offender and victim, only the offender, and only the victim were habitual drinkers; 13.2% of the victims were alcoholics. Most of those killed by a spouse, parent, or descendent were also alcoholics. In 1962, 17% of the rape victims were intoxicated—10.7% slightly, 5.4% moderately, and 1.3% severely. (RUCAS)

2. Incest

335. Awad, G. A. Father-son incest: A case report. *The Journal of Nervous and Mental Disease,* 1976, *162,* 135–139.

A case of father-son incest is presented. The sexual involvement occurred while the father was intoxicated and, as he reported later, unaware of his behavior. Investigation of the family interrelationships revealed numerous difficulties involving the wife's passivity, the adolescent son's delinquency, and the husband's unconscious struggle with homosexual impulses, which he attempted to deny with various behavioral expressions of virility and authority. The father, a heavy drinker, considered his son's acting-out behavior a challenge to his authority and masculinity; alcohol influenced the breakdown of his ego controls during the incidents. Treatment consisted of conjoint marital therapy in which the husband's abstinence was a primary goal. (RUCAS)

336. Browning, D. H., & Boatman, B. Incest: Children at risk. *American Journal of Psychiatry,* 1977, *134,* 69–72.

The typical family constellation in this study of 14 cases of incest was that of a chronically depressed mother, an alcoholic and violent father or stepfather, and an eldest daughter who was forced to assume many of her mother's responsibilities, with ensuing role confusion. The authors stress the need for physicians to be alert to the possibility of incest in such high-risk families. (RUCAS)

337. Dogliani, P., & Micheletti, V. Sull'influsso della intossicazione alcoolica acuta nell'incesto e nella zoofilia. [On the influence of acute alcohol intoxication on incest and zoophilia.] *Rivista Spermentale di Freniatria e Medicina Legale delle Alienazioni Mentali,* 1958, *82,* 485–499.

Five cases are reported in which men, in states of acute intoxication, committed incest or sodomy. The nature of the effects of alcohol is discussed, and literature is cited on sexual deviations. It is concluded that the abnormal behavior described is a result of the depressant action of alcohol on the frontal lobes, which control the behavior of man with respect to the outside world. (RUCAS)

338. Gross, M. Incestuous rape: A cause for hysterical seizures in four adolescent girls. *American Journal of Orthopsychiatry,* 1979, *49,* 704–708.

Four cases of hysterical seizures in adolescent girls (mean age 14) raped by fathers or father surrogates are discussed. All of the men were alcoholics and committed the rapes when drunk or during alcoholic blackouts. (RUCAS)

339. Meiselman, K. C. Participants in father-daughter incest. In K. C. Meiselman, *Incest: A psychological study of causes and effects with treatment recommendations.* San Francisco, CA: Jossey-Bass, 1978.

Characteristics of father and daughter incest participants are described and discussed as they have been revealed in previous studies, and as they appeared in case histories. Reference is made to alcoholism and alcohol abuse as lowering inhibitions among the fathers, permitting behavior that would be suppressed in a state of sobriety. (NCALI)

340. Merland, A., Fiorentini, H., & Orsini, J. A propos de 34 expertises psychiatriques se rapportant a des actes d'inceste pere-fille. *Annales de Médecine Légal,* 1962, *42,* 353–359. (Cited in N. Lukianowicz, Incest: I. Paternal incest, *British Journal of Psychiatry,* 1972, *120,* 301–313.)

Of 34 cases of father-daughter incest, alcoholism was found in 10 fathers and serious psychiatric disturbances in 22. (Author)

341. Phillip, E. La personnalité des délinquants d'inceste. *Acta Medicinae Legalis et Socialis (Liege),* 1966, *19,* 199–201. (Cited in N. Lukianowicz, Incest: I. Paternal incest, *British Journal of Psychiatry,* 1972, *120,* 301–313.)

More than 50% of 182 incestuous fathers were alcoholics, and a great number were "imbeciles." (Author)

342. Scripcaru, G., Pirozynski, T., & Parus, N. Considérations sur certains aspects médico-légaux et psychiatriques de la délinquance sexuelle. *Acta Medicinae Legalis et Socialis (Liege),* 1966, *19,* 175–181. (Cited in N. Lukianowicz, Incest: I. Paternal incest, *British Journal of Psychiatry,* 1972, *120,* 301–313.)

In 2 cases of paternal incest both fathers had suffered from alcoholic encephalopathy with atrophy of the frontal lobes. (Author)

343. Szabo, D. Problemes de socialisation et d'integration socio-culturelles: Contribution a l'etiologie de l'inceste. [Problems with socialization and socio-cultural integration: Contribution to the etiology of incest.] *Canadian Psychiatric Association Journal,* 1962, *7,* 235–249.

This is a sociological study based on 96 well-documented cases of father-daughter incest from the files of the Department of Health in Montreal between 1937 and 1954. Cases chosen for study were those with the most complete records. Examination of family structure and situation did not reveal any particular factor relating to occurrence of incest. In some cases the incest barrier was not well established or socialization was such that the abnormal was considered normal. In other situations there were predisposing factors: absence of the wife, provocative attitude of the daughter, alcoholism, and father's depression.

344. Virkkunen, M. Incest offences and alcoholism. *Medicine, Science, and the Law,* 1974, *14,* 124–128.

Clear differences were found between alcoholic and other incest offenders in a study of psychiatric records at the Helsinki University Central Hospital for the period 1945 to 1972. The alcoholic group showed more evidence of previous criminal offenses, particularly acts of violence, and had more often exhibited aggression at home prior to the detection of incest. The spouse had a rejective sexual attitude toward the offender in alcoholic cases more frequently than in other cases. There was also evidence that the alcoholic offender was more often under the influence of alcohol at the beginning of the relationship; incest was more often reported in those cases involving alcoholic offenders; and fear of the alcoholic offender often resulted in concealment of the incestual relationship by the spouse or the victim. It is concluded that the release of inhibitions generally attributed to alcohol is a major contributing factor in cases of incest involving alcoholic persons.

345. Weinberg, S. K. *Incest behavior.* Secaucus, NJ: The Citadel Press, 1955.

This book views incest as an extreme form of deviant behavior, a sign of family disorganization, and a condition that has serious effects on the personality development of the youngster involved in incestuous relationships. Approximately 200 cases of incest that came to the attention of the authorities were studied to understand the family, personality processes, and settings in which the incest behavior took place. Alcoholism was seen as a contributor to incestuous behavior by contributing to a decline in general responsiveness to social constraints. A typical male incest partner, brother or father, characteristically has a history of arrests for personal offenses such as drunkenness, wife-beating, or bigamy; rarely are there histories of property offenses. When alcohol is used to alleviate inner disturbances, such as feeling irritable, depressed, and quarrelsome, the distress may be relieved but the person becomes more sexually excited. There are many who commit incest when intoxicated but refrain when sober.

3. Child Molesting

346. Aarens, M., Cameron, T., Roizen, J., Roizen, R., Room, R., Schneberk, D., & Wingard, D. *Alcohol, casualties and crime.* (Report No. C-18, Selected studies on the societal-epidemiological aspects of alcohol use and alcohol-related problems.) Berkeley, CA: National Institute on Alcohol Abuse and Alcoholism, November 1977.

This is an extensive review which includes a section on sexual abuse of children. Incidence of child molesting is difficult to determine. Official statistics vary considerably over time and with geographic location. The statistics appear to reflect the degree of concern with the problem more than actual prevalence. Problems with operational definitions and legal definitions create confusion in differentiating exhibitionism, statutory rape, and child molesting. Studies are almost always based on child molesters confined to mental hospitals or prisons. Empirical data reveal a considerable degree of variation in alcohol involvement. In the 11 studies examining alcohol involvement at the time of the offense, percentages ranged from 19% to 49%. Percentages in 18 studies examining the incidence of a history of drinking problems among child molesters ranged from 7% to 52%. Alcoholism is evidenced in a disproportionately high number of child molesters, compared to prison controls, particularly heterosexual offenders who use force or threat. Incest offenders are characterized by a larger proportion of both alcoholics and offenders who were drinking at the time of the offense when compared with other child molesters. (NCALI)

347. McCaghy, C. H. Drinking and deviance disavowal: The case of child molesters. *Social Problems,* 1968, *16,* 43–49.

Of 158 men convicted of sexually molesting a child under 14 years of age, 51 admitted the crime and implicated alcohol as a cause (group A), 78 admitted the crime but did not mention drinking (group B), and 29 denied committing the offense (group C). To compare the 3 groups, 133 of the 158 were asked to speculate on the motives of other child molesters:

49% of group A, 68% of group C, but only 30% of group B attributed derogatory motives, which suggests that neither the "deniers" nor the "drinkers" identified with other child molesters. More in groups A and C suggested punitive treatment for other child molesters than in group B (30%, 47%, and 16%, respectively). If therapy aims at making offenders accept full responsibility for their crimes, success should be reflected in greater tolerance of other offenders. Among patients in group A, 64% of those who attended 20 or fewer sessions, but only 35% of those who attended more than 20 sessions attributed derogatory motives to other child molesters; in group B, 38% and 24%; and in group C, 67% and 70%. This indicates that therapy is less successful with the deniers. The data suggest that as long as offenders can maintain a normal self-image through displacement of blame onto alcohol, they are essentially similar to deniers (group C). It is suggested that the disavowal of deviance acts as a self-corrective device, serving to forestall future deviance, and that forcing the offender to accept the label of deviant may serve to maintain rather than eliminate a pattern of deviant behavior. (RUCAS)

348. Rada, R. T. Alcoholism and the child molester. *Annals of the New York Academy of Sciences*, 1976, *273*, 492–496.

A strong association between drinking, alcoholism, and child molestation was observed in a study of data on 203 pedophilic sex offenders committed to Atascadero State Hospital, California. Forty-nine percent of the child molesters were drinking, and 34% were drinking heavily (10 or more beers or the equivalent), at the time of the offense. The alcoholism rate for the group was 52%, based on results of the Michigan Alcoholism Screening Test (MAST), while 33% were alcoholic according to Pokorny's Shortened MAST. A significantly lower incidence of drinking at the time of the offense was observed in male-child molesters than in female-child molesters. In addition, the male-child molesters had a definitely higher alcoholism rate than the female-child molesters. The importance of these findings for treatment programs is emphasized.

349. Swanson, D. W. Adult sexual abuse of children. *Diseases of the Nervous System*, 1968, *29*, 677–683.

Twenty-five consecutive cases of sexual offense against a minor, referred by the courts for psychiatric evaluation, were reviewed. Subjects were between the ages of 18 and 67 with a mean age of 33. Half of the subjects consumed alcohol to excess; 28% were severe alcoholics. Many had history of sexual deviation (24%) or had achieved inadequate adult heterosexual adjustment (56%). Some subjects willingly admitted to excessive use of alcohol or exaggerated their alcohol intake in an apparent effort to minimize personal responsibility for the act. In one-third of the offenders heavy alcohol intake preceded the offense and seemed to contribute significantly to the deviant behavior. In most cases involving alcohol, the offender behaved with consistently poor judgment, even when sober, e.g., history of promiscuity or vagrancy. In other cases, use of alcohol combined with loss of usual source of sexual gratification led to an impulsive act of sexual deviancy.

350. Whitfield, C. L. Children of alcoholics: Treatment issues. *Maryland State Medical Journal*, 1980, *29*, 86–91.

The special problems of the children of alcoholics and their treatment are reviewed. The problems include child abuse and neglect, hyperactivity, behavior and school problems, suicide, chemical dependency, depression, sexual adjustment, and functional illness. It is essential to treat the children with the parents and to recognize that their family's problem is alcoholism. The nonalcoholic parent should attend Al-Anon; pre-Alateen and Alateen could be beneficial for the children. When they grow into adults, they should attend Al-Anon or similar treatment groups. Denial and ignorance are cited as the major reasons for inappropriate treatment. Remedial steps include caregivers' playing the proper role model, education of health professionals, screening of parents, confronting the family with the problem, offering hope, empathizing, using employee assistance programs, and publications of observations in journals. (RUCAS)

4. Miscellaneous

351. Allen, D. M. Young male prostitutes: A psychosocial study. *Archives of Sexual Behavior*, 1980, *9*, 399–426.

A 3-year study of male prostitutes is presented with relevant data about their origin, their social and family background, education, sexuality, drug and alcohol use, and delinquency. A classification has been developed which separates the male prostitutes into 4 groups: (1) full-time street and bar hustlers, (2) full-time call boys or kept boys, (3) part-time hustlers, usually students or employed, and (4) peer-delinquents, who use prostitution and homosexuality as an extension of other delinquent acts (assault and robbery). Similarities and differences between the 4 groups in terms of their psychosocial background, motives, and type of operation are described. Limited follow-up data indicate that only part-time male prostitutes, who continue in education or vocational training, have a reasonable expectation of an eventually stable social adjustment. (Author)

352. Apfelberg, B., Sugar, C., & Pfeffer, A. Z. A psychiatric study of 250 sex offenders. *American Journal of Psychiatry*, 1944, *100*, 762–770.

The material for this study was obtained by analyzing the clinical records of 250 nonpsychotic male sex offenders who were examined in the psychiatric division of Bellevue Hospital. Moderate to excessive use of alcohol was reported by 91 (39%) of the subjects; 61 (25%) denied any use of alcohol; 66 (27%) admitted occasional drinking.

353. Banay, R. S. Alcoholism and crime. *Quarterly Journal of Studies on Alcohol*, 1942, *2*, 686–716.

This study examines the relationship between alcoholism and the criminal activities of more than 3,000 inmates in Sing Sing Prison between 1935 and 1940. Subjects were divided into 2 groups: intemperates, whose alcoholism appeared before persistent commission of crimes; and controls, who were nondrinkers or whose alcoholism was subsequent to their criminal lifestyle. Psychiatric evaluation found more psychopathology among the intemperates than the controls. The crimes of the intemperates, who represented 25% of the total sample, were judged to be alcohol related or the direct result of alcohol intoxication. The following types of crimes are most prevalent among those early in their alcoholism who, without criminal records prior to their becoming alcoholic, commit series of diversified, serious crimes: absurd and irrational crimes, sexual crimes, and crimes of acquisitive nature. After confirmed intemperance, chronic alcoholics commit the following crimes: irresponsible acts of no criminal significance, foolish and mischievous acts (joy rides), and poorly planned acquisitive crimes with very meager results. Serious crimes, such as the following, are committed when intoxicated: atrocities, sexual crimes, and violent crimes.

354. Bartholomew, A. A. Alcoholism and crime. *Australian and New Zealand Journal of Criminology,* 1968, *2,* 70–99.

The relationship between alcoholism and crime was studied by examining the frequency of chronic alcoholism and of being under the influence and drinking near the time of the crime in male prisoners serving sentences of 3 months or more. Types of crime were offenses against property, aggressive offenses, sexual offenses, and miscellaneous. Alcohol was a factor in between 39.2 and 52.8% of the different types of sexual cases.

355. Bell, R. R. Prostitution. In R. R. Bell, *Social deviance: A substantive analysis.* Homewood, IL: Dorsey, 1971.

The history of prostitution is traced, discussing the sociocultural forces shaping its function as a social institution. Prostitutes of lesser status sell themselves directly on the street or in bars. Higher status prostitutes, call girls, usually avoid bars and make contact with customers through pimps or referral by other call girls. Some call girls work cocktail lounges. Many lounges encourage call girls because they increase business. Prostitution is analyzed as a subculture with particular demographic characteristics, folklore, and myths. These are described and discussed in detail.

356. Blane, H. T. Middle-aged alcoholics and young drinkers. In H. T. Blane & M. E. Chafetz (Eds.), *Youth, alcohol, and social policy.* New York: Plenum, 1979.

It is argued that there are 2 "alcoholisms": one referring to traditional clinical, diagnostic and treatment nomenclature, the other to the transitory social and behavioral consequences of "frequent heavy drinking" (episodic consumption of relatively large amounts of alcohol on a single occasion). The latter clusters in adults aged 18–24, especially men. Analysis of national databases indicates that, for problems directly attributable to alcohol, middle-aged men and women have higher rates than young adults for liver cirrhosis mortality,

inpatient and outpatient care episodes for alcohol abuse, and arrests for drunkenness. Young adults have higher rates for drunken driver mortality and arrests for driving while intoxicated and liquor law violations. Young adults have higher rates than middle-aged adults of motor vehicle and other accident mortality, divorce, arrests for disorderly conduct, vandalism, serious crimes against persons, other assaults, rape, sex offenses, prostitution and commercialized vice, and offenses against family and children. These findings suggest that the social and human costs associated with alcoholism, on the one hand, and problems stemming from frequent heavy drinking, on the other, probably do not differ greatly. (RUCAS)

357. Bowman, K. M. Some problems of addiction. In P. H. Hoch & J. Zubin (Eds.), *Problems of addiction and habituation.* New York: Grune & Stratton, 1958.

Many addictive substances and related problems are addressed in this chapter. One of these is alcoholism and homosexuality, sexual deviance, and crime. Changes in attitude are traced from the earlier, punitive attitudes to more enlightened, accepting positions held by legal, religious, and medical professionals in recent years.

358. Cruz, J. C. Criminogenia sexual y algunas consideraciones médico-legales. [Sexual criminogenesis and other medical-legal considerations.] *Revista Mexicana de Psiquiatrica Neurologia,* 1943, *10,* 3–14.

Among 744 delinquents studied at the Institute of Criminology, 86 were sexual delinquents. The type of crime, education, occupation, economic status, etc., of the subjects are presented. The role of alcohol in the 86 sexual crimes is as follows: 37 delinquents (46.8%) were constant drinkers, 15 delinquents (18.9%) were drunk at the time of committing the crime, and 27 (34.5%) were nondrinkers. In the first group (constant drinkers), alcohol cannot be the determining factor in the commission of the crime because it lowers potency; but other psychopathological elements may explain the crime. In the second group (occasional drinkers), alcohol may be responsible for the commission of the crime because of its immediate aphrodisiac action and its effect on the central nervous system and sexual glands. In the third group, some physical or psychopathological defect must have been responsible, not alcohol. (RUCAS)

359. De Vito, R. A., & Marozas, R. J. The alcoholic satyr. *Sexuality and Disability,* 1981, *4,* 234–245.

Satyriasis is an extremely rare disorder characterized by uncontrolled sexual hyperactivity in males who have little or no capacity for deep emotional involvement. Four case histories are presented and discussed in terms of psychodynamic processes underlying the disorder. Three of the 4 cases were encountered in a population of 1,200 alcoholics attending 2 alcoholism treatment centers in Chicago within a span of 2 years. The fourth had presented himself to an outpatient mental health clinic in the same geographical area requesting treatment for homosexuality; he was also found to abuse alcohol. Satyriasis is conceived of as "sexual addiction." Among the 2 cases for whom alcohol abuse was diagnosed an addiction, interest in sex and ability to perform was significantly diminished with increased alcohol use. After a brief abstinence from alcohol, however, the "sexual addiction" reappeared. The condition is attributed to both psychodynamic and biological processes.

360. Division of Alcohol Rehabilitation, State of California Department of Public Health. *Criminal offenders and drinking involvement: A preliminary analysis* (Publication No. 3). Berkeley, CA: Author, 1960.

The study population consisted of 2,325 newly committed male felons. Of these, 98% used alcohol and 52% had been arrested at some time on drinking charges. Half of the subjects who drank claimed to have consumed alcohol before committing the crime for which they were sent to prison and 29% claimed to have been intoxicated. The highest proportions of those who reported drinking before the crime were in categories of crimes of violence and crimes against persons, e.g., sex crimes, murder, and assault. Of the sex offenders, 38% reported being intoxicated at the time of the offense.

361. Flaxman, N. Nymphomania—A symptom: Part II. Psychoses. *Medical Trial Technique Quarterly,* 1973, *19,* 305–316.

This article examines nymphomania as a symptom of serious psychiatric disorder. Among the disorders discussed is toxic psychosis induced by alcohol. The author observes that the chronic alcoholic is more likely to be a prostitute than a nymphomaniac.

362. Gebhard, P. H., Gagnon, J. H., Pomeroy, W. B., & Christenson, C. V. *Sex offenders: An analysis of types.* New York: Harper & Row; Paul B. Hoeber, Inc., Medical Books, 1965.

Data were gathered between 1940 and 1960 through interviews conducted primarily in Indiana and California. Three groups of White males comprise the subjects of the study: the sex-offender group, 1,356 males convicted for one or more sex offenses; the prisoner group, 888 males convicted for a serious offense other than a sexual offense; and the control group, 477 males never convicted for offenses more serious than traffic violations. Sex offenders were classified by characteristics of the offense (i.e., gender of the offended person, age of the offended one, relationship of the offended to the offender, involvement of force, and involvement of physical contact), and classes of offenders were compared to the prisoner and control groups on a variety of dimensions of sexuality, e.g., masturbation, sex dreams, and homosexual activity. Nonsexual factors contributing to or related to the offense are examined as well, including use and abuse of alcohol. Alcohol is discussed as a causative factor in 2 ways: (1) personality deterioration from alcoholism leading to criminal lifestyles, and (2) regressive behavior and disinhibition resulting from acute intoxication. Intoxication is associated with legally punishable behavior but does not appear to determine the form of the behavior. Both the sex offender and the prisoner groups used alcohol significantly more than did the control group. Alcohol is discussed in chapters devoted to particular classes of offenses, in a discussion of the setting of the offense, in a chapter on miscellaneous factors, and in the chapter on sexual psychopaths.

363. Glover, J. Notes on an unusual form of perversion. *International Journal of Psychoanalysis,* 1927, *8,* 10–24.

This case study presents an in-depth analysis of a 35-year-old alcoholic man with a complex shoe fetish. The fetish involved a rigid, intricate ritual for obtaining the shoes and achieving orgasm. The woman selected met precise criteria: she was from his social class, drank moderately, and wore high-heeled shoes of particular styles and colors. She would be taken to dinner and encouraged to over-indulge in alcohol to the point of staggering. Drinking alcohol had conscious sexual significance and watching a woman drink aroused him sexually. Once the desired level of the woman's intoxication was reached, he took her into the open air to walk until exhausted and falling. He would remove her shoes and, after observing a compulsive ritual in arranging the shoes, he masturbated to scenes from dinner. The psychodynamic processes and psychosexual development issues determining this behavior are discussed in detail.

364. Glueck, B. C., Jr. *Final report: Research project for the study and treatment of persons convicted of crimes involving sexual aberrations, June 1952 to June 1955.* Albany, NY: New York State Department of Mental Hygiene, 1956.

Three groups of prisoners incarcerated in Sing Sing Prison between 1952 and 1955 were subjected to psychiatric evaluation: sex offenders, 170 men who had been convicted of sex crimes, e.g., rape, sexual assault, incest; offender controls, 50 men convicted of aquisitive or violent crimes; and Negro offenders, 51 men differing from the offender controls only by race (both the sex offender and offender control groups contain Blacks and Whites). The sex offenders were found to be more disturbed than the controls. Alcoholism was found at a rate of about 50% among sex offenders and controls and 40% among the Blacks. Drinking began earlier for the sex offenders; 66% began before age 25, compared to 52% of the controls and 27.5% of the Blacks. Moderate to severe alcohol intoxication was present at the time of the crime in 44% of the sex offenders. The sex offenders were found to be generally lacking in control and judgment, and alcohol may have contributed to the event by further impairing controls and judgment. Sexual offenders were grouped into 8 categories that could be differentiated behaviorally and by offender characteristics. Alcohol intoxication or alcoholism figured prominently only for offenders who committed rape or sexual assault on an adult female. The rapist was more likely than other offenders to commit the offense when self-control was diminished by alcohol. Rapists, more than any other offender groups, were likely to report sexual arousal as an effect of alcohol. Alcoholism was a prominent feature among offenders committing rape (60% of rapists were moderate to severe alcoholics), heterosexual abuse of an adolescent female (57% were alcoholics), and incest (70% of incest offenders were alcoholics).

365. Gromska, J., Smoczyński, S., & Bardzik, S. Przypadek aktu nekrofilii dokonanego w upojeniu patologicznym. [A case of necrophilia committed in a state of pathological intoxication.] *Psychiatra Polska,* 1969, *3,* 207–209.

366. Haberman, M. A., & Michael, R. P. Autocastration in transsexualism. *American Journal of Psychiatry,* 1979, *136,* 347–348.

Historically, autocastration has been associated with psychosis or psychotic reactions while intoxicated. It had been noted that amputation of the testes, in contrast to other self-inflicted injuries, gave both satisfaction and relief and was not regretted. Transsexualism has since emerged as a distinct diagnostic entity and transsexual patients are able to obtain medically sanctioned surgery for what, in the past, had been self-inflicted with the assistance of alcohol. Two case histories of autocastration are presented. For anesthesia, one patient injected lidocaine into the skin of the scrotum and the other drank a quantity of alcohol. Both performed careful self-surgery. After disposing of the testes, both obtained medical aid. Each demonstrated strong feminine identification and physical repudiation of their male genitalia. Neither was psychotic at the time of the autocastration and psychiatric deterioration did not follow.

367. Henn, F. A., Herjanic, M., & Vanderpearl, R. H. Forensic psychiatry: Profiles of two types of sex offenders. *American Journal of Psychiatry,* 1976, *133,* 694–696.

The authors examined records of 239 individuals charged with sexual offenses and referred by the courts to a forensic service. Defendants charged with rape were typically under 30 and had histories of antisocial behavior that included other types of violence. Major mental illness was rare in this group. Child molesters in the sample were of no particular age, usually had no history of violent behavior, and had a low incidence of psychosis. The most common secondary diagnosis for both rape and child molestation was alcoholism and drug abuse, constituting one-third of the secondary diagnoses for the 2 groups. (Author)

368. Hoppe, H. *Alkohol und kriminalität.* [Alcohol and criminality.] Wiesbaden: J. F. Bergmann, 1906.

369. Huszár, I., & Gabor, I. Quelques aspects médico-légaux actuels de l'alcoolisme chronique. [Some current medicolegal aspects of chronic alcoholism.] *Annales de Médecine Légale,* 1966, *46,* 5–11.

Among the crimes committed by 202 alcoholic persons in Hungary were 3 homicides, 19 assaults, and 9 sexual offenses.

370. Huszár, I., & Irányi, C. Problémes relatifs aux delits d'ordre sexuel commis sous l'influence de l'alcool. [Problems relating to sexual offenses committed under the influence of alcohol.] *Annales de Médecine Légale,* 1966, *46,* 255–261.

Sexual offenses (homosexuality, gerontophilia, fetishism) committed while intoxicated by 3 male unskilled laborers, ages 24 to 38, are reported. It is stressed that sexual anomalies that arise only under the influence of alcohol may constitute a special form of atypical intoxication and consequently must be judged as such. In a first offense, it constitutes a factor that excludes or limits responsibility; if repeated, the offender must be held responsible. (NCALI)

371. Irányi, J., & Somogyi, E. Voyeur magatartás és módosulása szokvany részegségben. [Voyeuristic behavior and its variations in common drunkenness.] *Orvosi Hetilap,* 1979, *120,* 1885–1888.

Cases of 3 voyeurs who always drank before committing the offense are described. In a 57-year-old man who was a moderate drinker, the voyeurism was associated with coprolagnia, and post-mortem analysis (he drowned in the excrements of an outhouse) revealed a blood alcohol concentration of 0.24%. A 29-year-old man, who led a drunken and irregular life and had undergone alcoholism treatment, drank about one liter of wine and 5 beers before the act (he climbed ladders and electric poles apparently unimpaired by alcohol), while a 21-year-old voyeur and exhibitionist with a similar lifestyle usually drank 7-8 beers before the act, but did not feel too drunk and remembered all the details (he climbed to the roof of a 4-story house and descended via the lightning rod). (RUCAS)

372. Irányi, J., & Somogyi, E. Das voyeur-verhalten und dessen modifizierung unter alkoholeinfluss. [The voyeur behavior and its modification under the influence of alcohol.] *Psychiatrie, Neurologie und Medizinische Psychologie,* 1980, *32,* 199–205.

This is a German translation of an article originally published in Hungarian (see entry 371). (RUCAS)

373. Lenoir, L. Alcool et criminologie. [Alcohol and criminology.] *Lille Medical,* 1980, *25,* 160–163.

The association between crime and blood alcohol concentrations (BAC) in criminals and their victims is examined. It is important to know the BAC of criminals at the time the crime was committed to determine responsibility. Alcohol can cause a temporary loss of responsibility and rationality. In 78% of 82 criminal offenses studied, the aggressor or the victim or both were intoxicated (BAC>0.08%); in 16% only the victim was intoxicated; in 17% only the aggressor; and in 45% both victim and aggressor. The possible role of alcohol in encouraging vulnerable behavior is briefly discussed, and alcohol's effect on psychological processes is mentioned. (RUCAS)

374. Lésniak, R., & Szymusik, A. Orzecznictwo sadowo-psychiatryczne w przestepstwach seksualnych. [Forensic psychiatric expertise in sexual offenses.] *Psychiatria Polska,* 1978, *12,* 245–251.

375. McGeorge, J. Alcohol and crime. *Medicine, Science and the Law,* 1963, *3,* 27–48.

Two main groups of alcohol-related crime are distinguished: those resulting from the effects of alcohol and those in which alcohol itself is the motive. In the first group, in New South Wales (year not stated), there were 5,095 cases of driving under the influence and 69,259 cases of being drunk and disorderly. Many of the 14,433 cases of riotous, offensive, and indecent behavior owe their origin to excessive indulgence. To the second group belong the "grogsellers" (433 cases) and Liquor Act violators (2,678 cases). The relationship between alcohol and juvenile crime is reviewed, citing investigators early in this century. In English and Australian law, drunkenness is not generally regarded as an aggravation of crime and may operate to reduce punishment. Over a 3-year period, 22 of 85 murderers in New South Wales were "addicted to drink," as were the offenders in 59 of 100 assault and robbery cases, 598 of 1,221 breaking, entering, and stealing cases, 46 of 340 false pretenses cases, and 96 of 425 sex offenders against females. In the same period, of 2,171 persons arrested for serious crimes, 821 had a history of heavy drinking. The incidence of driving "under the influence" is increasing, and this may be related to increased alcohol consumption. Literature is reviewed regarding offenses in which alcohol is a factor, and some statistics are cited from various sources which indicate that homicide related to sexual jealousy is the most common and characteristic form of alcoholic crime with conscious motive. Sexual offenses are also strongly related to the use of alcohol. In crimes of acquisition alcohol is more often the motive than the cause. Alcohol is a dangerous stimulant to psychopaths, overthrowing the little control they have. Total prohibition, however, is considered undesirable. (RUCAS)

376. Mohr, J. W., Turner, R. E., & Terry, M. B. *Pedophilia and exhibitionism.* Toronto: University of Toronto Press, 1964.

This book explores the nature of 2 forms of sexual behavior which represent the majority of sexual offenses coming to the attention of the courts. The material presented is the result of studies conducted at the Forensic Clinic of the Toronto Psychiatric Hospital, established to assist the courts in the assessment and treatment of offenders. Combining all studies, a total of 247 sex offenders were studied. The sample included those convicted for rape, indecent assault, indecent exposure, gross indecency, indecent acts, or contributing to juvenile delinquency. Subjects were diagnosed as pedophiles, exhibitionists, and homosexuals. Among younger offenders (those under 40), alcoholism does not appear to play a significant role, although some offenders may be intoxicated at the time of arrest and may report that they were drinking at the time of the offense. Occurrence of sexual offenses, particularly exhibitionism, among older offenders tends to occur in connection with chronic alcoholism and organic deterioration.

377. Murphree, H. B. Addiction and sexual behavior. In R. Slovenko (Ed.), *Sexual behavior and the law.* Springfield, IL: Thomas Books, 1965.

The common conceptions of the laity about drug addictions are highly inaccurate. Addicts themselves are a poor source of information about addiction, because they are often as superstitious and suggestible about drug effects as other laypersons. In some cases, their psychopathology colors their imaginations even more floridly than that of their more well-adjusted contemporaries. Indeed, the very definition of what constitutes addiction is not clear, because it tends to be influenced by what the public disapproves of rather than by more objective criteria. Among the ideas widely entertained is the assumption that there is some intimate relationship between drug addiction in some forms and sexual activities, especially those of a perverse or licentious nature. This probably plays an important part in the rather unreasoning revulsion the public often demonstrates toward these forms of addiction. This irrationality is made more poignant by the fact that addiction to other agents, such as alcohol, which is far more destructive both to the individual and to society, is generally tolerated with minimal sanctions by the public. The object of this chapter is to evaluate the effects of the more frequently misused drugs upon sexual physiology and to attempt to reconcile these with what is known of the emotional disturbances of addicts of all kinds. (Author)

378. Nichols, F. L., & Haines, D. The difficulties of dual denial in the treatment of sex offenders with alcoholism. *International Journal of Offender Therapy and Comparative Criminology,* 1979, 23, 214–220.

Based on treatment experience at a psychiatric center in British Columbia, Canada, the interrelated synergistic action between alcoholism and sexual offenses and the similarities between alcoholics and sex offenders are discussed. Partly because of the stigma attached, both tend to delude themselves and others about their affliction and to rationalize and deny it. The usefulness of Alcoholics Anonymous programs in treating sex offenders who are alcoholics and the usefulness of having acknowledged sex offenders in treatment programs for this population are pointed out. The role of alcohol and other drugs, and that of early maladjustments and psychological instability in making persons alcoholics and sex offenders, and the problems of treatment are discussed. (RUCAS)

379. Otto, S. Single homeless women and alcohol. In Camberwell Council on Alcoholism, *Women and alcohol.* New York: Tavistock Publications, 1980.

The alcohol problems of women alcoholics in the United Kingdom who are not part of an intact family, and who regularly use cheap rented accommodations, are described. Those who have become involved in the penal system (e.g., convicted of prostitution, larceny, police assault, etc.) are distinguished from those who have not. Both groups require consideration because (1) the powerful environmental factors that shape lives in this distinct skid row subculture should be studied; (2) drunkenness in women seems to upset people more than drunkenness in the homeless per se or in men alcoholics, and these attitudes influence the provisions made for them; and (3) the common assumption that the problems of homeless alcoholic women are the same as those of men should be challenged. There are enough homeless women and women living in skid row accommodations to warrant attention, particularly since this population has more physical and psychiatric problems than their counterparts in common lodging houses and hostels. It is also likely that alcohol problems are prevalent in women who have been banned from lodging houses, even though they have gone undetected because it is assumed that alcoholism is the prerogative of men. (RUCAS)

380. Piotrowski, Z. A., & Abrahamsen, D. Sexual crime, alcohol, and the Rorschach test. *Psychiatric Quarterly Supplement,* 1952, *26,* 248–260.

Of 100 imprisoned sex offenders studied, 58 were intoxicated at the time their crime was committed. Rorschach tests were administered to test the hypothesis that if a person's *M* responses (human movement) are more active and expansive than *FM* responses (animal movement), s/he is likely to behave with more restraint under alcohol and more likely to commit a crime while sober, and vice versa. The comparative quantity and quality of the M and FM responses were correlated with the state of the offender's inebriation at the time of the crime. The proposed correlation between Rorschach responses and inebriation/sobriety was observed in 84 persons.

381. Power, D. J. Sexual deviation and crime. *Medicine, Science and the Law,* 1976, *16,* 111–128.

The various types of sexual deviation and their treatment are discussed, and relevant case histories are presented. It is noted that a potential sex criminal may become an active one as the result of ingesting alcohol or taking illicit drugs, especially in cases of rape and incest. (RUCAS)

382. Prus, R., & Irini, S. *Hookers, rounders, and desk clerks: The social organization of the hotel community.* Toronto: Gage, 1980.

This book represents a participant-observer study about "hookers" (prostitutes) and strippers, bartenders and cocktail waitresses, bar patrons, and "rounders" (persons engaged in illegal activities), who together form the "hotel community" subculture. (RUCAS)

383. Rada, R. T., Kellner, R., Laws, D. R., & Winslow, W. W. Drinking, alcoholism, and the mentally disordered sex offender. *Bulletin of the American Academy of Psychiatric Law,* 1978, *6,* 296–300.

The prevalence of alcoholism and degree of drinking at the time of the offense were studied in 382 mentally disturbed sex offenders committed to Atascadero State Hospital (CA); 53% of all offenders (including child molesters, rapists, incest offenders and exhibitionists) were drinking at the time of the offense. Most of them (46–69%) reported drinking heavily. The Michigan Alcoholism Screening Test identified 50% of offenders as alcoholics. More alcoholics than nonalcoholics (81% vs. 25%, p < .005) were drinking at the time of their offenses. Sex offenders may need alcoholism treatment. (RUCAS)

384. Rada, R. T., Laws, D. R., & Kellner, R. Plasma testosterone levels in the rapist. *Psychosomatic Medicine,* 1976, *38,* 257–268.

The reported relationship between testosterone level and both sexual and aggressive behavior suggested this study of the testosterone level in rapists, since rape is an offense that ostensibly combines aggressive and sexual behavior. Plasma testosterone was measured in 52 rapists and 12 child molesters who had completed the Buss-Durkee Hostility Inventory, the Megargee Overcontrolled Hostility Scale, and the Michigan Alcoholism Screening Test. The rapists were classified according to the degree of violence during the commission of the rape. The ranges and means of the plasma testosterone levels for the rapist and child molester controls were within normal limits. The group of rapists who were judged to be most violent had a significantly higher mean plasma testosterone level than normals, child molesters, and other rapists in this study. Alcoholic rapists had a significantly higher mean plasma testosterone level than nonalcoholic rapists. Mean Buss-Durkee hostility rating scores for rapists were significantly higher than the mean for normals, but there was no correlation between individual hostility scores and plasma testosterone levels. There was no correlation between age, race, or length of incarceration and plasma testosterone level. (Author)

385. Ramee, F., & Michaux, P. De quelques aspects de la délinquance sexuelle dans un département de l'ouest de la France. [Some aspects of sexual offenses in a province in western France.] *Acta Medicinae Legalis et Socialis,* 1966, *19,* 79–85.

Of 480 criminal offenses reported in a province in western France, 106 were sexual offenses, of which 34 occurred under the influence of alcohol. Of the latter, 13 were incestuous. First offenses occurred when girls reached age 10 and were repeated with the same or other children in the family. Alcoholism, particularly prevalent in western France, is discussed as a responsible factor. The apparent passiveness of wife and daughters is mainly due to fear of violence and fear of losing the breadwinner in case of detention. The importance of prevention is emphasized; improvement in the rural environment, education, and an anti-alcoholism campaign are urgently recommended. (RUCAS)

386. Ribeiro, A. L. Medico-legal aspects of alcoholic intoxication. *Medico-Legal Journal,* 1963, *31,* 95–99.

In this presidential address to the Medico-Legal Society of Kenya, the author addresses the medico-legal aspects of alcoholic insanity. There are 4 specific alcoholic insanities: delirium tremens, acute confusional insanity, Korsakov's disease, and alcoholic dementia. In delirium tremens are restlessness, irritability, and vivid, terrifying hallucinations associated with tremor. The patient may become violent and homicidal and may attempt suicide to escape the hallucinations. Korsakov's disease is a type of alcoholic insanity associated with severe peripheral neuritis. It results in loss of memory for recent events and extreme dissociation. In acute confusional insanity, hallucinations occur which are less terrifying than those of delirium tremens. The patient becomes active and grandiose; some cases have delusions of persecution. The most prominent feature of alcoholic dementia is loss of memory and the habit of supplying blanks in memory by the fabrication of events that have not occurred. When sexual crimes, assault, and homicide arise from hallucinations and trivial events being interpreted to support delusional beliefs, the criminal cannot be held responsible for his/her acts. In addition, crimes are committed "under the influence of drink," which may mitigate the court's decisions on punishment. In such cases, the only reliable evidence is blood or urine analysis.

387. Rommeney, G. Ungewöhnliche formen des alkoholrausches. [Unusual forms of alcohol intoxication.] *Deutsche Zeitschrift für Gerichtliche Medizin,* 1952, *41,* 277–288.

Pathological intoxication is usually diagnosed as such only when violent actions expressive of primitive drives are apparent. Finer signs of unusual or abnormal intoxication are considered normal without referring them to the usual behavior of the individual in question. Many of the finer aberrations are as important psychopathologically as the expansive obvious actions. Several cases are presented to illustrate. Unusual intoxication can occur in psychically stable persons. A temporary intolerance to alcohol may take place in a stable person who has been subjected to unusual and stressful circumstances, such as war, disappointment in love, or exhaustion. Sexual crimes committed under the influence of alcohol particularly evidence the fact that intoxication is an exogenous vegetative disturbance of regulatory mechanisms and must be regarded in the same way as other diseases of the diencephalon with psychic symptoms. Reactions vary not only from individual to individual but within the same person. The psychotic expansion under the influence of alcohol is not limited to criminal acts of violence. Every state of intoxication that develops in an unpredictable fashion, the kind of reaction depending on the magnitude of the vegetative disturbance of the regulatory mechanism, should be recognized as abnormal and pathological in a broader sense. (RUCAS)

388. Safko, S., & Stancak, A. Vztah alkoholu k sexuálnej delikvencii. [Alcohol and sexual delinquency.] *Casopis Lékaru Ceskych,* 1980, *119,* 494–496.

The authors analyzed the behavior of 179 delinquents prosecuted for sexual offenses with a particular view to the ingestion of alcohol at the time of the offense, as well as to the possible diagnosis of chronic alcoholism in the offenders. Ninety-eight delinquents (57.4%) committed criminal offenses in alcoholic intoxication. The drinking of alcohol was found to have been the salient feature in the criminal offense of rape (81%) and incest (66%). Chronic alcoholism was diagnosed in 40 offenders (22.3%). Having compared their notes with literary data, the authors reached the conclusion that the abuse of alcoholic drinks is a significant criminogenic factor in relation to sexual delinquency. (English abstract and English title were provided as a summary at the end of foreign article cited above.) (Author)

389. Selling, L. S. The role of alcohol in the commission of sex offenses. *Medical Record,* 1940, *151,* 289–291.

An analysis of 100 consecutive cases of male sex offenders was made to determine what role, if any, alcoholism had in the commission of the offense. The offenders could be separated into 3 groups on the basis of the way in which alcohol was used. The first group, 8% of the total, consisted of chronic alcoholics. The members of this group had deteriorated so greatly that they lacked insight into the social significance of their acts. They were not particularly disturbed over their offenses, and their conduct was probably a chance relationship motivated by lack of inhibitory mechanisms rather than caused by any characteristic psychopathic drive. The second group, 35% of the total, consisted of men who were not chronic alcoholics but who had been drinking at the time the offense was committed. These occasional drinkers were probably escaping from an intolerable situation which was set up by the complexes that lead to a latent desire for sexual misbehavior. Inhibitory mechanisms were temporarily broken down; the offenders admitted they could not commit their offenses when sober and their records tended to prove these statements. The third group, 57% of the total, consisted of men who were sober when the crime was committed. This group comprised every type of psychopathology. More frank psychopathology was found in it than among the previous group. There were a number here who showed no frank abnormality of any kind. (RUCAS)

390. Takman, J. Promiskuosa, prostituerade och alkoholiserade flickor? [Promiscuous, prostituted and alcoholic girls?] *Sociale Meddelelser,* 1962, 389–398.

The records of 94 young prostitutes in Stockholm disclosed that 35 were misusers of alcohol, 23 of them since before prostitution.

391. Topiar, A., & Vilc, M. Zoofilní aktivity v alkoholickém opojení. [Zoophilic activities during alcohol intoxication.] *Protialkoholický Obzor,* 1980, *15,* 33–35.

Two cases of men who engaged in zoophilic activities while intoxicated are described. Alcohol probably stimulated what could have been latent zoophilia. Both men were married and had normal sexual lives. (RUCAS)

392. Wagner, K. Alkohol und sexualdelikte. [Alcohol and sexual offenses.] *Kriminalbiologisch Gegenwartsfragen,* 1964, *6,* 93–100.

Most sexual crimes are determined by the personality structure of the criminal, and often the role of alcohol is secondary. Effects of different amounts of alcohol on the commission of crimes and the problem of mitigation are discussed. (RUCAS)

393. Wilschke, K. Über die kriminogene rolle des alkohols bei sittlichkeitsdelikten. [The criminogenic role of alcohol in sex offenses.] *Munchener Medizinische Wochenschrift,* 1965, *107,* 176–177.

Among the 442 sex offenders arrested during 1957–1963, 20% were under the influence of alcohol at the time of the crime. This includes only those cases in which the intoxication was ascertained by witnesses or by chemical tests. In 18% of the cases the offenders were alcoholics and in 3% they had previously been indicted for offenses committed during intoxication. Among the 276 child molesters 19% were under the influence of alcohol at the time of the offense and 12% were alcoholics. It is no longer believed that alcohol plays a dominant role in sex offenses. More stress is laid on the instinctive drive. (RUCAS)

B. Venereal Disease

394. Adler, M. W. Diagnostic treatment and reporting criteria for gonorrhoea in sexually transmitted disease clinics in England and Wales. *British Journal of Venereal Diseases*, 1978, *54*, 15–23.

Investigation of gonorrhea treatment methods in England and Wales showed that in 152 (89%) of 171 clinics for men and in 132 (76%) of 173 clinics for women the consultants asked the patients to refrain from drinking alcohol during treatment. The most common reasons given were that alcohol irritates the urethra and increases the severity of symptoms (48%), that patients should remain sober to lessen sexual intercourse resulting from intoxication (28.2%), that restraint from drinking lessens relapse and post-gonococcal urethritis (26.3%), and that alcohol delays drug absorption (12.2%). Some practitioners admitted that they advocated cessation of drinking because it is standard practice (16%) but that they were not sure it was of any use. (RUCAS)

395. Akimochkina, R. G., & Derbinskaya, G. M. [The role of alcoholism in dissemination of venereal diseases.] *Vestnik Dermatiologii I Venerologii* 1978, *4*, 40–43.

Based on the analysis of questionnaires from patients with venereal diseases, the role of alcoholism in the dissemination of these diseases was demonstrated. In order to control the dissemination of venereal diseases, venereologists should know the syndromes of alcoholism. It is necessary to solve the problem of simultaneous treatment of venereal diseases and alcoholism. (English abstract and English title were provided as a summary at the end of foreign article cited above.) (Author)

396. Arya, O. P., Alergant, C. D., Annels, E. H., Carey, P. B., Ghosh, A. K., & Goddard, A. D. Management of non-specific urethritis in men. *British Journal of Venereal Disease*, 1978, *54*, 414–421.

A trial comparing the efficacy of 3 different tetracyclines, each in 2 different dosage regimens, in the treatment of nonspecific urethritis is described. There was a significant association between the retreatment rate and sexual intercourse. Abstinence from alcohol is recommended as it appears that alcohol contributes to the rate of unprotected intercourse, leading to the need for retreatment. Age, race, duration of symptoms, previous infection, and indulgence in alcohol did not appear to influence the results, whereas treatment of sexual contacts before resumption of sexual intercourse significantly reduced the retreatment rate. Single-dose treatment with doxycycline was shown to be ineffective. Treatment with doxycycline for 7 days or triple tetracycline for 7 days was less effective than triple tetracycline for 21 days or oxytetracycline for 7 or 21 days, all of which gave the same success rate. (Author)

397. Chuchelin, G. N., & Sluchevskaia, M. P. Epidemiologicheskaya rol' lits, zloupotreblyayuschikh alkogolem, v rasprostranenii venericheskikh zabolevanii. [Epidemiological role of persons who misuse alcohol in the spread of venereal diseases.] *Vestnik Dermatiologii I Venerologii*, 1978, *4*, 43–46.

The role of alcohol abuse in the dissemination of venereal diseases is discussed, and the correlation between prevalence of alcoholism and of venereal diseases is pointed out. Thus, in 1975, the region of Bryansk had 2.7 times fewer registrations for alcoholism per 100,000 population than was the average for the whole republic, and the occurrence of syphilis was 3.3 times and that of gonorrhea 2.6 times lower than the republic's average. Further, a study is described in which 2 groups of patients with venereal diseases (number and age not stated) were compared: (1) a group of alcohol abusers who were as a rule intoxicated during sexual intercourse, and (2) a group of infrequent drinkers who were sober during sexual contacts (controls). More of the male and female alcohol abusers than male and female controls had secondary syphilis (men, 20% vs. 16%; women, 51% vs. 33%), a past history of gonorrhea (2 and 6 times more men and women, respectively), and contracted the disease from casual partners (syphilis: 52% vs. 21%, and 38% vs. 9.4%; gonorrhea: 60% vs. 25%, and 40% vs. 12%). The alcohol abusers also have 2 or 3 times more frequently waited over 1 month after the first symptom before contacting the physician. (RUCAS)

398. Hart, G. Social aspects of venereal disease: II. Relationship of personality to other sociological determinants of venereal disease. *British Journal of Venereal Disease*, 1973, *49*, 548–552.

This study investigates the relationship of personality to sociological parameters associated with venereal disease infection (i.e., age, education, and socioeconomic status). The author hypothesizes that certain personality types, comprised of high extraversion and high neuroticism, are prone to behaviors generally recognized as antisocial (including alcohol abuse) which result in greater exposure to venereal disease. The Eysenck Personality Inventory and a sociological questionnaire were completed by 206 servicemen, then analyzed for sociological and personality differences. The main findings were: (a) extraversion and neuroticism decreased with age; (b) higher neuroticism was associated with lower social status and less education; and (c) increasing extraversion was associated with increasing alcohol intake, civil arrests, and military charges. Comparisons between these results and studies associating extraversion with venereal disease patients and antisocial behavior such as excessive alcohol consumption lead the author to conclude that his hypothesis is supported.

399. Medhus, A. Venereal diseases among female alcoholics. *Scandinavian Journal of Social Medicine,* 1975, *3,* 29–33.

The incidence of gonorrhea among 71 female alcoholics was studied from the twentieth year before to the ninth year after the first compulsory treatment by the Temperance Board of Malmo. Twenty-five subjects had, at some time, had gonorrhea. The mean age at the first infection was high, over 28 years. Nonetheless, the onset of gonorrhea was an early "symptom." Recorded criminal offense, receipt of public assistance, and conviction for drunkenness usually appeared later. Each individual's risk of contracting gonorrhea was assessed from tabulated data concerning the gonorrhea incidence among Malmö women in general, specified by calendar year and age. A total of 53 infections was observed, as against 6.9 expected. The ratio of observed to expected gonorrhea was not particularly high in the early period of observation. From the twelfth year before up to one year before the first compulsory treatment, the ratio increased to roughly 15 to one. This high ratio remained during the subsequent years. Syphilis was diagnosed in 5 subjects. (Author)

400. Medhus, A., & Hansson, H. Alcohol problems among female gonorrhoea patients. *Scandinavian Journal of Social Medicine,* 1976, *4,* 141–143.

The subject group consists of 286 women who, in 1960, were treated for gonorrhea in the Out-patient Clinic for Venereological Diseases in Malmö. During the years 1932 to 1973, they were responsible for 119 convictions for drunkenness, the expected number of convictions being 4, as calculated from an age and calendar year specific risk table for Swedish women. The difference between numbers observed and those expected increased with age. Of the 82 patients aged 25 years or over in 1960, one in 10 had previously been convicted for drunkenness; 13 years later the ratio was one in 7. During the years 1939 to 1973, 12 gonorrhea patients were subjected to compulsory treatment by the Temperance Boards. Of the patients aged 25 years or over in 1960, one in twenty had earlier been subjected to such treatment; 13 years later it was one in ten. It is concluded that gonorrheal infections, particularly in women 25 years and over, can constitute a "symptom" of alcohol problems. (Author)

401. Schofield, C. B. S. Psychological and sociological considerations. In J. Money & H. Musaph (Eds.), *Handbook of sexology.* New York: Excerpta Medica, 1977.

This chapter addresses psychological and sociological considerations in the acquisition and transmission of venereal disease. One of the factors contributing to the increase in venereal disease is alcohol abuse. Previous findings reveal a high proportion of men and women who contracted venereal disease had met in a bar or had been to a bar before having sexual intercourse. In the military, higher rates of venereal disease are found among servicemen who drink heavily. Alcohol becomes a factor in venereal disease in that it facilitates sexual intercourse with casual acquaintances.

402. Schofield, C. B. S., Wilson, E., Patel, A. R., McGhie, T., & Wilson, G. M. Blood ethanol concentrations in patients attending special clinics in Glasgow. *British Journal of Venereal Disease,* 1975, *51,* 340–344.

This study was prompted by previous findings suggesting an association between heavy drinking or alcoholism and the contracting of sexually transmitted diseases. Blood samples for measurement of ethanol concentrations were taken from 543 male and 158 female patients who were having serological tests for syphilis at the Special Clinics in Glasgow, Scotland. Ethanol was detected in 56 men and 8 women. It is assumed that the subjects' blood alcohol levels at the time of attending the clinic represented an index of the subjects' usual alcohol consumption. However, psychological and sociological factors are believed to influence the data for this sample. For instance, male patients attending the clinic for the first time had the highest incidence of detectable blood alcohol. Drinking before attending the clinic is attributable to the stress of the event. An example of a sociological factor is a Wednesday afternoon peak in incidence of detectable blood ethanol corresponding to attendance at a football match, which is locally associated with drinking before, during, and after the match. Among women, the highest incidence occurred among promiscuous women who had been visiting bars as part of their regular activity. Those with the highest concentrations were unreliable attenders, often not completing the course of treatment.

403. Sushchenko, L. V., Borovik, V. Z., & Shraiber, V. G. Sluchai gigantskikh gangrenoznykh iazv u bol'nykh vtorichnym sifilisom. [Giant gangrenous ulcers in secondary syphilis.] *Vestnik Dermatiologii I Venerologii,* 1979, *6,* 71–74.

A case is reported of a 40-year-old unmarried, promiscuous woman with secondary syphilis who developed 2 giant gangrenous ulcers at the sites of syphilitic elements (hard chancres or erosive papules) and an ulcer in the small pudential lip leading to perforation of the lip; the woman was an alcoholic, which might have contributed to the extremely rare complication. (RUCAS)

404. Wells, B. P. W., & Schofield, C. B. S. "Target" sites for anti-V.D. propaganda. *Health Bulletin,* 1970, *28,* 75–77.

The authors believe a close association between alcoholism and promiscuity has been established. Furthermore, they assert that promiscuous sexual behavior is associated with incidence of venereal disease. They suggest that posting warning notices and information on the prevention of venereal disease in select locations would ensure that education attempts would be directed where they would be most effective. In order to pinpoint the best locations for distribution of V.D. warnings, information was taken from the files of V.D. clinics in Glasgow, Scotland, on 496 males who acquired V.D. from a partner other than their wives. Information consisted of where they met their infected consort and where the infection was subsequently acquired. Public houses were the commonest meeting place, reported by 35.1% of the subjects, this being most commonly reported by older men: 55% of men aged 40–49, and 75% of those over 50. The second most common meeting place was dances, 30.6% overall, particularly among the young: 36% of young men aged 10–19, 36.9% of those aged 20–29, and 30.6% of men aged 30–39.

C. Alcoholism and Homosexuality

1. Both Sexes (or Gender Unspecified)

405. Alcoholics Anonymous World Services, Inc. *Do you think you're different?* New York: Author, 1976.

This pamphlet contains 13 stories of men and women whose race, age, sexual preference, or social status deviate from the stereotype associated with A.A. members and alcoholics in general. These stories illustrate how A.A. can help a broad spectrum of people achieve sobriety. Two homosexuals, a man and a woman, describe how they came to A.A., their early misgivings about A.A., and how they finally found A.A. to be helpful in their struggle with alcoholism.

406. Beaton, S., & Guild, N. Treatment for gay problem drinkers. *Social Casework*, 1976, *57*, 302–308.

This article deals with the treatment of gay individuals, both male and female, through group counselling. Although the group described dealt with individuals with alcoholic problems, the authors hope that such group methods can be employed with gay people having other problems. To date there have been few, if any, articles in the literature reporting on work with gay people who have alcohol or other problems in a group setting with male and female gay members and "straight" male and female co-leaders. The group experience discussed here led the authors to question the applicability of many of the studies that have reported gay people to be difficult to work with, particularly in a group setting. It appears, from the authors' experience, that, if trust can be established between straight therapists and gay clients, then group treatment can offer an effective and efficient mechanism to assist gay individuals to the same degree as such treatment assists heterosexual individuals. Additionally, the authors believe that the lack of success of many group treatment attempts with gay clients has been due to limiting their emphasis to the problems of being gay or to changing their sexual preference, rather than emphasizing the total problems which led clients to request help. (Author)

407. Chemical Dependency Program. *A counselor's guide to the special needs of sexual minority clients in alcoholism and drug treatment.* Seattle, WA: Author, 1980.

Special social, cultural, and emotional factors contribute to a high rate of alcoholism within the gay population. The gay bar is the primary setting for socializing. Alcohol and drug use constitute an important part of social activity for gay men and lesbians. Social condemnation and contempt severely limit homosexuals' alternatives for socializing or recreation.

Self-hate, guilt, and shame contribute to the development of addictions since alcohol and drugs offer the best relief available for these feelings. The gay alcoholic or drug abuser may be unable to obtain help for several reasons: (1) services are denied by agencies who feel they are not geared to handle homosexual clients' needs, (2) homosexuality is often seen as the cause, and therefore, sexual orientation, not the alcoholism, is the object of treatment, (3) silence about sexual preference is required, (4) care givers often overreact to displays of affection or dress, and (5) patronizing or overly indulgent attitudes are taken toward homosexuality. Specific suggestions are made for counsellors suggesting ways in which they can assist gay clients in revealing their sexual orientation and their special needs. Guidelines for counsellor's responses to the revelation are also presented. These can be summarized as a call for: (a) treating the gay client with respect and dignity, (b) being prepared with resource material, e.g., information on Gay A.A. groups, and (c) honestly assessing personal attitudes towards homosexuality and how they may affect service delivery.

408. Fenwick, R. D. Alcohol and other drugs. In R. D. Fenwick, *The advocate guide to gay health*. New York: E. P. Dutton, 1978.

In this chapter, statistics are reported indicating that one in 3 members of the gay community is, or is well on the way to becoming, an alcoholic. It is suggested that alcoholism exists to the extent it does because of gay bars. That is, patrons go to bars for the opportunity to meet friends, not to drink, but they end up drinking quite frequently. It is pointed out that the lesbian subculture is not noticeably bar-oriented and that homosexuality outside of the bar setting must also be considered. The psychological and physiological relation between alcohol and sexuality is discussed.

409. Fifield, L. *Alcoholism and the gay community*. Paper presented at the National Council on Alcoholism Annual Meeting, Seattle, May 1980.

Some of the problems that are unique to the gay community in the development of alcoholism and alcohol abuse are addressed. The author explores gay and nongay alcoholism treatment program approaches toward the problem of gay alcoholism and offers some insight as to why there is such a high incidence of alcohol abuse within the gay community. Factors that contribute to the excessive use of alcohol are enumerated, and the responsibilities of the gay community and the larger nongay community in dealing with these issues are outlined. (NCALI)

410. Finnegan, D. G., & McNally, E. B. *Alcoholism, recovery, and health: Lesbians and gay men*. Paper presented at the National Council on Alcoholism Annual Meeting, Seattle, May 1980.

The author contends that almost everyone raised in the American culture learns negative attitudes toward homosexuals and that changing those attitudes is a long and difficult process. This process of unlearning and relearning that the alcoholism professionals need to engage in if they wish to deliver high quality treatment to the recovering gay male and/or lesbian alcoholic is described and discussed. The following topics are examined: (1) current definitions of health and the development of a more inclusive definition; (2) special needs, issues, and problems of recovering gay males and lesbians; (3) facets of lesbian and gay male lifestyles which the professional needs to learn about; and (4) special role of the openly gay and/or lesbian alcoholism professional in helping colleagues and clients to know that lesbians and gay men are healthy too. (NCALI)

411. Fox, V. *Special treatment problems: The homosexual alcoholic*. Paper presented at the Utah University School on Alcoholism and Other Drug Dependencies Workshop, Salt Lake City, June 1980.

Special treatment problems associated with homosexual alcoholics are discussed. (NCALI)

412. Freudenberg, H. J. The gay addict in a drug and alcohol abuse therapeutic community. *Homosexual Counseling Journal*, 1976, *3*, 34–45.

The experience of the gay individual within a therapeutic community is examined from 2 perspectives: the gay person who admits to being gay and the gay person who cannot admit to being gay while in the therapeutic community. Gay addicts and alcoholics who do not admit to being gay are living a continuous lie during their stay in the treatment facility. They face a double-pronged problem of breaking away from their addiction and simultaneously hiding their gayness or defending themselves against undercurrents of prejudice against gays. When the addict or alcoholic is a woman, there is a third problem. She must contend with being a woman in relation to a predominantly male staff. Most therapeutic communities are run by straight men from racial minority groups who have unresolved sexual and role identity problems they have brought with them from the outside society. Many staff members and residents will respond to a resident who admits to being gay with ridicule, discrimination, and verbal assault. The gay residents who are hiding their gayness may resort to the manipulative behavior they are being encouraged to abandon in order to get along and to demonstrate their progress. There is a need for openness among straight staff members and a realignment of their attitudes so that they can provide open, accepting role models for all residents. There is also a need for treatment facilities to employ gay staff members or gay consultants to provide gay residents with role models for entering a drug-free, gay world.

413. The Gay Community Services Center. *On my way to nowhere—alienated, isolated, drunk: An analysis of gay alcohol abuse and an evaluation of alcoholism rehabilitation services for the Los Angeles gay community*. Los Angeles, CA: Author, 1975.

This report summarizes the results of a survey of the gay community with regard to drinking behavior, problems unique to the gay alcoholic, and alcoholism treatment services for gay alcoholics in the Los Angeles area. The study finds a strong relationship between alienation and alcohol abuse. Limited social options for gay people have contributed to a prevalent reliance on bars for socializing and meeting friends, and the setting itself contributes to high rates of alcohol consumption. Bar users average 6 drinks per night, frequenting bars on an average of 19 nights per month. Gay alcoholics are in need of comprehensive services including hot lines, counselling, group meetings, employment aid, justice system assistance, and social activities, provided in a supportive atmosphere with peer contact in the recovery process. The 3 gay agencies in the Los Angeles area were evaluated and found to meet high standards of service delivery successfully but to lack the resources to serve a community as large as that of the Los Angeles area. Of the 46 nongay agencies surveyed, 43 treat gay clients rather than refer them to gay agencies. A general lack of services specific to gay people was found. For instance: only 2 agencies have group therapy specifically for gay clients, no agencies provide nontherapy groups for their gay clients, and only 3 of 35 agencies providing couples counselling have same-sex couples in the program. In addition, nongay agencies do not provide an atmosphere where gay people, staff or clients, can comfortably reveal their gayness.

414. Gay Council on Drinking Behavior, Whitman-Walker Clinic, Inc. *The way back: The stories of gay and lesbian alcoholics*. Washington, DC: Author, 1981.

As an introduction to this book, some common reasons given by gay and lesbian persons for drinking and distressing problems that may occur because of drinking are described. Ten true accounts of the lives of gay and lesbian alcoholics who reached a point where alcohol was controlling their lives are presented. It is stated that there is a way to build a new constructive life of infinite possibilities without alcohol for most gay alcoholic men and women, primarily by the removal of alcohol through the Alcoholics Anonymous program. (NCALI)

415. Jones, K. A., Latham, J. D., & Jenner, M. D. *Social environment within conventional alcoholism treatment agencies as perceived by gay and non-gay recovering alcoholics: A preliminary report*. Report presented to the National Council on Alcoholism Annual Meeting, Seattle, May 1980.

A preliminary report of the Orange County (CA) Gay Alcoholic Needs Assessment Project, reported to the National Council on Alcoholism Convention (Seattle, Washington, May 3, 1980), is presented. Sexual preference as a personal background variable was isolated and an attempt was made to assess its effect on patient-program interaction. Using the COPES (Community-oriented Programs Environment Scale), differences in perceived social environment within recovery facilities, as experienced by gay and nongay recovered alcoholics, were examined. Results of profile scores indicate that both groups want much of the same thing from a treatment environment, that is, a program that places strong emphasis on the relationship dimension and that has a personal problem orientation. Gay subjects reportedly wanted more emphasis on staff control. In reference to the controversy of whether gays should be treated in their own separate facilities, only about half chose to go to all-gay facilities. Nevertheless, they also wanted not to hide the gay part of their identity. An outline of COPES subscales and definitions is appended. (NCALI)

416. Judd, T. D. A survey of non-gay alcoholism treatment agencies and services offered for gay women and men. In D. E. Smith, S. M. Anderson, M. Buxton, N. Gottlieb, W. Harvey, & T. Chung (Eds.), *A multicultural view of drug abuse: Proceedings of the National Drug Abuse Conference, 1977*. Cambridge, MA: Hall & Co.; Schenkman Publishing Co., 1978.

A survey of 57 nongay treatment agencies in the San Francisco Bay area revealed: (1) the traditional attitudes of alcoholism agency staff toward women's sex roles are strongly correlated with a negative attitude toward lesbians and gay men, (2) the traditional attitudes toward men's sex roles are strongly correlated with negative attitudes toward lesbians, (3) a strong correlation exists between authoritarianism among agency staff and negative attitudes toward lesbians and gay men, and (4) alcohol agency staff hold more traditional attitudes, are more authoritarian, and hold more negative attitudes toward lesbians and gay men than gay service organization staff. It is concluded that nongay alcohol treatment agencies do not meet the primary needs of the gay and lesbian alcoholic for they fail to address the special needs of gays/lesbians and to provide a supportive, accepting atmosphere in which clients can deal with their problems.

417. Lolli, G. Alcohol and homosexual behavior. In G. Lolli, *Social drinking: The effects of alcohol*. New York: Collier Books, 1961.

Homosexuality is seen as the result of early childhood experiences and permissive attitudes toward adult homosexual behavior. The relationship between homosexuality and excessive drinking can take 3 forms as follows: (1) open homosexual behavior exhibited during temporary sobriety, (2) homosexuality revealed only during drinking episodes, or (3) homosexual behavior occurring both in sobriety and inebriety. In the author's opinion, adequate treatment of the alcoholic homosexual calls for treatment of both the excessive drinking and the homosexuality.

418. Loucks, C. C., & Higgins, G. J. *The gay alcoholic: A problem of parallel stigmas*. Paper presented at the National Conference on Alcoholism Annual Meeting, Seattle, May 1980.

It is contended that homosexuality and alcoholism are stigmas in society. The gay male alcoholic has 2 stigmas: homosexuality and alcoholism. The lesbian alcoholic has 3 stigmas: being a woman, homosexuality, and alcoholism. The external attitudes of society toward homosexuality and alcoholism are identified and defined. Solutions are also identified, defined, and proposed for the internalized attitudes of the individual gay male or lesbian alcoholic. It is concluded that there is a need to confront societal attitudes regarding homosexuality and alcoholism and that education is a formidable tool for this task. It is also concluded that acceptance of homosexuality or alcoholic identity by the homosexual individual initiates a process that frees his/her internally stigmatized state and that such groups as Alcoholics Anonymous (A.A.) and gay A.A. groups are necessary support systems for this process. (NCALI)

419. Marcelle, G. *Alcoholism and the gay community: The state of knowledge today*. Paper presented at the Third National Lesbian and Gay Health Conference, San Francisco, June 1980.

Societal attitudes toward alcoholism and homosexuality are briefly discussed. It is emphasized that until 1979 a "wall of silence" among health care professionals, especially within the alcoholism field, remained largely intact surrounding the subject of gay alcoholism. In 1979, an informal gathering of gays attended the Rutgers Summer School of Alcohol Studies, which led to the founding of the National Association of Gay Alcoholism Professionals (NAGAP). One of the NAGAP accomplishments was their assistance to the National Council on Alcoholism (NCA) in coordinating a 2-day track on alcoholism and the gay community for NCA's 1980 Forum, which was held in Seattle, Washington. Papers presented at this forum on gay alcoholism are cited and discussed. It is concluded that during this forum 2 concepts repeatedly surfaced: (1) that there is an urgent need for much more research into gay alcoholism and for written program models, particularly ones based on the success of those few already in operation, and (2) that most of the needs of the gay alcoholic population are likely to be met only by the gay community itself. (NCALI)

420. Marden, P. G. *Prevalence of alcohol abuse in the gay population of the United States*. (Report No. RPO 310.) Canton, NY: St. Lawrence University, Department of Sociology and Anthropology, January 1980.

In this report an attempt is made to estimate the prevalence of alcohol abuse among the homosexual population of the United States by correlating available data on homosexuality rates and alcohol abuse rates in the general population, and by considering such factors as the singular importance of the bar culture and related drinking patterns in gay culture. Establishing a definitive rate proved difficult because both alcoholism and homosexuality are considered deviant behaviors by society at large and as such are often hidden. While the distinction between the "unacknowledged" and "acknowledged" homosexual groups and the supporting contention from Kinsey that sexual preference is a continuum do provide a way of dealing with the potential clientele for various services, including those that are alcohol related, little information is available on the size of either group. A tentative conclusion is that one in every 3 acknowledged homosexual encounters problems with beverage alcohol. It is suggested that those interested in alcohol abuse by gays develop their own estimates based on local circumstances, but do so with the expectation of careful evaluation. Recommendations for further research are offered. (NCALI)

421. Marschall, R. *Homosexual, alcoholic group therapy: A specialized treatment.* Paper presented at the National Council on Alcoholism Annual Meeting, Seattle, May 1980.

An overview of the relationship of the homosexual, the homosexual alcoholic, and the alcoholic to society is presented. The creation of a homosexual alcoholic group in a New York City hospital's alcoholism clinic is discussed. Difficulties encountered in the formation of this group and specific treatment goals are also discussed. It is concluded that the homosexual alcoholic group can effectively help this population to adjust to the general stresses of integrating into society as sober persons, and at the same time begin to face internalized homophobia, which is a hidden and often unrecognized enemy and threat to the maintenance of sobriety. (NCALI)

422. McKaen, M. *Sexual minority service agencies in the eighties: Where do we go from here?* Paper presented at the National Conference on Alcoholism Annual Meeting, Seattle, May 1980.

The closing address of the sexual minority track of the 1980 National Conference on Alcoholism is presented. The influence of the nation's economy during the 1980s on the role of the sexual minority human service agencies is discussed. (NCALI)

423. Michael, J. *The gay drinking problem . . . there is a solution.* Minneapolis, MN: CompCare Publications, 1976.

In this pamphlet the author offers a personal discussion of life as a homosexual who is also an alcoholic. Along with his own story, he discusses the definition of alcoholism, who is an alcoholic, the progressive stages of alcoholism, the value of sobriety, detoxification, and relapse. The pamphlet concludes with descriptions of information and support organizations for alcoholics, with emphasis on services for gays.

424. Michael, J. *Sober, clean & gay!* Minneapolis, MN: CompCare Publications, 1977.

This pamphlet presents a discussion of recovery from alcoholism from the perspective of the sober gay alcoholic. The author speaks from personal experience as he discusses the need for honesty and changes in attitude, how to deal with homophobia, sexuality and sobriety, and the spiritual issues important to the alcoholic who is also gay. A guide to resources for gay alcoholics is provided.

425. Mongeon, J. E., & Ziebold, T. O. *Preventing alcohol abuse in the gay community: Towards a theory and model.* Paper presented at the National Council on Alcoholism Annual Meeting, Seattle, May 1980.

Major components of a prevention model for the gay community are described. The approach is grounded in the belief that, for an alcohol-abuse prevention program to be successful with a particular community, it must be sensitive to the values and norms of that community, be conducted by trusted and visible community members, involve a broad spectrum of the community leaders and opinion makers in its planning and implementation, and be integrated into the existing institutions and service delivery networks within that community. An early intervention and outreach program for gay men and women identified as ''at risk'' with beverage alcohol is proposed. The intervention component consists of an intensive, experimental group process that will encourage participants to develop more constructive alternative behavior in their lives. It is proposed that this intervention effort be accompanied by a public education and/or outreach campaign. It is suggested that the formal and informal communications networks of the gay community be utilized, and that the effort involve broad community representation in order to heighten gay awareness of the destructive consequences of alcohol misuse and to develop additional alternative outlets exclusive of ''bar and brunch'' activities. (NCALI)

426. Nardi, P. M. *Co-alcoholism in the non-traditional ''family'' structure of gays and lesbians.* Paper presented at the meeting of the National Council on Alcoholism Annual Meeting, New Orleans, April 1981.

Various family systems in which gay and lesbian people exist and how these relate to drinking behavior and its treatment and prevention are examined. A sociological perspective is used, emphasizing the values, norms, and meanings of drinking behavior in gay and lesbian communities. It is noted that this paper does not discuss all gay people; rather, it focuses on 2 types: those problem drinkers who are single yet active in a gay community and those who are committed to another person and identify themselves as part of a couple. (NCALI)

427. National Association of Gay Alcoholism Professionals. *NAGAP bibliography: Resources on alcoholism and lesbians/gay men.* Oakland, NJ: Author, 1980.

This bibliography provides a listing of materials on alcoholism and lesbians and/or gay men. The bibliography is divided into the following 3 sections: (1) a listing of resources that deal specifically with alcoholism and lesbian and/or gay men, (2) materials helpful to understanding lesbians and/or gay men and their culture, concerns, and lifestyles, and (3) additional resources on alcoholism. (NCALI)

428. Newmeyer, J. A. The sensuous hippie part II: Gay/straight differences in regard to drugs and sexuality. *Drug Forum*, 1977, *6*, 49–55.

Questionnaire data from 19 male and 11 female homosexuals were compared with data from 40 male and 25 female heterosexuals. Homosexuals hold more libertarian attitudes toward sexual activity in general. They are more likely then heterosexuals to use drugs to enhance sex, favoring alcohol as a sexual enhancer more than heterosexuals. However, 50% of all groups reported enjoying sex more while intoxicated.

429. Saghir, M. T., & Robins, E. *Male and female homosexuality: A comprehensive investigation.* Baltimore, MD: Williams & Wilkins, 1973, 119–120; 277–279.

Alcohol use and abuse as well as beliefs about the effects of alcohol on sexual behavior are surveyed among 89 male homosexuals, 35 male heterosexuals, 57 female homosexuals, and 43 female heterosexuals. Female heterosexuals reported least incidence of excessive drinking or alcohol dependence (5%) compared to female homosexuals (35%), male homosexuals (30%), and male heterosexuals (20%). Female heterosexuals were most likely to report that alcohol in moderate amounts enhances sexual experiences (56%), compared to 29% of heterosexual males, 22% of homosexual females, and 15% of homosexual males. Percentages reporting that alcohol use interferes with sexual functioning are also given: 2% of homosexual males, 12% heterosexual males, and 2% homosexual females; no percentage is given for heterosexual women. Homosexual males were far more likely than homosexual females to attribute problem drinking to their homosexuality.

430. Schofield, M. *Sociological aspects of homosexuality.* Boston: Little, Brown, 1965, 178–180.

The author argues against the association commonly made between homosexuality and antisocial behavior, including alcoholism. The homosexual lifestyle necessitates nonconformity but not necessarily antisocial attitudes.

431. Schwartz, L. R. *Alcoholism among lesbians/gay men: A critical problem in critical proportions.* (Report No. DIN 712.) Phoenix, AZ: Do It Now Foundation, 1980.

It is noted that data from a variety of sources placed the toll on alcoholism among sexual minority persons (lesbians and gay men) at between 20% and 32% of the gay population, with most reports finding that men and women are affected equally. The following topics in relation to alcoholism among lesbians and gay men are discussed: (1) the roots of the alcoholism epidemic, (2) changes in treatment agencies, (3) education of counselors, (4) 2 programs for sexual minorities and women, (5) gay groups of Alcoholics Anonymous, (6) organizing for the treatment of sexual minorities, and (7) the history of a popular lesbian feminist musician in her recovery from alcoholism. It is concluded that awareness is a vital key in approaching the current epidemic of alcoholism among sexual minorities and working toward prevention, and that an ultimate goal is to create an atmosphere in treatment facilities where openness is welcome and where gay staff members can in turn encourage their clients to feel comfortable in the treatment setting. A pamphlet entitled ''Alcoholism in the Lesbian/Gay Community: Coming to Terms with an Epidemic'' is provided. (NCALI)

432. Thomas, J. *A gay member's-eye view of Alcoholics Anonymous.* Paper presented at the National Council on Alcoholism Annual Meeting, Seattle, May 1980.

The author describes his personal experiences as a gay alcoholic in a nongay A.A. group and his subsequent joy in joining a gay A.A. group. The invitation to share no longer held the threat of exposure; gay A.A. members were not distracted from focus on recovery from alcoholism by disclosure of sexual orientation. Compassionate understanding without indulgence took shape in the context of gay and lesbian subculture, and a forum became available for talking about sex openly. Gay A.A. meetings provided an opportunity to let go of old ideas about gay life and to build a sense of ''family'' within the A.A. group. By providing the support of other gays and sober gay role models, gay A.A. makes a significant contribution to the gay community.

433. Wisconsin Clearinghouse for Alcohol and Other Drug Information. *Lesbians, gay men and their alcohol and other drug use: Resources.* Madison, WI: Author, 1980.

Recognizing that gay alcoholism is a problem, the Wisconsin Clearinghouse published this pamphlet, which annotates some of the few articles, pamphlets, and films available on this subject. The pamphlet was written for several diverse groups, including alcoholism counselors, members of the gay community concerned with this issue, and anyone interested in developing a better understanding of lesbians and gay men. (NCALI)

434. Ziebold, T. O. *Alcoholism and the gay community.* Washington, DC: Blade Communications, 1979.

This report describes the needs of gay alcoholics and treatment resources in the Washington, DC area. The incidence of alcoholism in the gay community is estimated to be significantly higher than among heterosexuals, particularly among gay women. Traditional social attitudes have stigmatized alcoholism and homosexuality, and psychiatrists have causally associated homosexuality with alcoholism so that the ''cure'' for alcoholism has been to ''cure'' homosexuality. The results have been tragic for gays. The stigma is ironically perpetuated by gay people who imagine that to admit to alcoholism would make them more of social outcasts. The above-average incidence of alcoholism among gays is believed to be related to the denial aspect of the illness. Gay men and women must build strong ego defenses to survive in our hostile society, which makes them vulnerable to addiction by blocking awareness of the growing dependency on alcohol. The gay community must accept responsibility for helping gay alcoholics. Settings for recovery should be provided within the gay community, and recovery should emphasize self-acceptance as a homosexual.

435. Ziebold, T. O. Ethical issues in substance abuse treatment relevant to sexual minorities. In D. J. Ottenberg & E. E. Madden (Eds.), *Ethical issues in substance abuse treatment: Proceedings of the 12 Annual Eagleville Conference, May 11, 1979.* Eagleville,

PA: Eagleville Hospital and Rehabilitation Center, 1980.

Gay men and lesbians recovering from chemical dependency have different issues and considerations to address in treatment. Addressing the whole person involves providing an opportunity for homosexuals to explore themselves in the context of their subculture, a subculture which is currently evolving new norms and is beginning to establish traditions. Our existing cultural heritage has created barriers to providing the comfort and support needed by homosexual clients to develop fully their identity as drug-free or alcohol-free individuals. This raises ethical issues for heterosexual service providers and calls for re-evaluation of their social values.

436. Zigrang, T. A. *Who should be doing what about the gay alcoholic?* Paper presented at the National Council on Alcoholism Annual Meeting, Seattle, May 1980.

Several studies have documented a 30% rate of alcoholism among homosexuals. Reasons cited for this high rate are reported, and the responses of alcoholism and gay counseling professionals to gay alcoholism are discussed. Treatment options for the gay alcoholic are examined with the conclusion that increased education for staff about the particular needs of the gay alcoholic and development of specialized services in existing treatment facilities are high priority. A description of the form of inservice training provided for one such staff and the results of such training are presented. Directions for future research in the area of gay alcoholism are suggested. (NCALI)

2. Females

437. Climent, C. E., Ervin, F. R., Rollins, A., Plutchik, R., & Batinelli, C. J. Epidemiological studies of female prisoners: IV. Homosexual behavior. *The Journal of Nervous and Mental Disease,* 1977, *164,* 25–29.

Study of 95 prisoners at the Massachusetts Correctional Institution for Women showed that the group of 27 heterosexuals scored higher on alcoholism than the 26 self-reported homosexuals and the 42 who were regarded as homosexuals by the prison staff (i.e., used homosexual behaviors as a means of adapting to the prison environment).

438. Diamond, D. L., & Wilsnack, S. C. Alcohol abuse among lesbians: A descriptive study. *Journal of Homosexuality,* 1978, *4,* 123–142.

Intensive interviews with 10 lesbian alcohol abusers were conducted to assess 4 theoretical causes of alcoholism: (1) gratification of dependency needs, (2) desire for enhanced power, (3) relief from stress related to sex-role expectations and conflicts, and (4) low self-esteem. Strong dependency needs, low self-esteem, and a high incidence of depression were revealed. Drinking increased power-related behaviors, enhanced self-esteem, and for many subjects increased feelings of depression. Findings suggest that lesbians with alcohol problems need therapists who will accept their sexual orientation, and treatment that will increase their sense of power and self-esteem without alcohol. Suggestions for future research are offered.

439. Dietrich, D. *Reaching out to the lesbian alcoholic.* Paper presented at the 1980 NCA Forum, Alcoholism and the Gay Community, National Council on Alcoholism Annual Meeting, Seattle, May 1980.

Alcoholism outreach methods targeting the lesbian population are outlined. Beginning from a nonjudgmental position, information on alcoholism and alcoholism treatment can be publicized in the media. Respected supporters and leaders of the lesbian community will disseminate information. Alternative routes such as sponsoring lesbian coffee houses, benefit concerts featuring feminist/lesbian entertainers, and consciousness raising groups can be useful in reaching alcoholic lesbians. In the lesbian community, word of mouth may be useful in spreading information about fair and supportive treatment services. Lesbian resource centers and lesbian/gay bars provide avenues for disseminating service information through announcements or posters.

440. Hawkins, J. L. Lesbianism and alcoholism. In M. Greenblatt & M. A Schuckit (Eds.), *Alcoholism problems in women and children.* New York: Grune & Stratton, 1976.

Comparing nonpatient lesbians with matched heterosexual controls, no significant differences in the prevalence of neurotic disorders was found, although there were more suicide attempts, more depression, and more alcoholism in the lesbian group. Findings are similar for gay men. In the area of alcoholism among gays, a notable absence of relevant literature reveals a lack of systematic research on the number of people in the gay community and the number of gay alcoholics. Studies that do exist focus on the Los Angeles area and are aimed at evaluating alcoholism treatment services available to gays. These studies report that traditional sex-role attitudes and negative attitudes toward homosexuality exist among treatment agency staff members and can interfere with adequate alcoholism treatment for gays. The author conducted an informal survey of 30 lesbian alcoholics, asking: (a) did lesbianism contribute to alcoholism and (b) should lesbian alcoholics be treated only by lesbian service providers? Twenty-eight of the women felt that lesbianism did not contribute to alcoholism; the other 2 were unsure. In response to the second question, all but 7 subjects, who were feminist lesbians, felt that treatment need not be delivered by another lesbian. The need for gay support was recognized. In the Los Angeles area, Alcoholics Together was founded by homosexual members of Alcoholics Anonymous.

441. Hogan, R. A., Kirchner, J. H., Hogan, K. A., & Fox, A. N. The only child factor in homosexual development. *Psychology, A Quarterly Journal of Human Behavior,* 1980, *17,* 19–33.

One hundred thirty-seven homosexual women who were only children, 68 homosexual controls who had siblings, and 47 nonhomosexual control subjects with only-child status were surveyed. The 3 groups were compared as to their attitudes and experiences in the areas of education, religion, family experiences, psychological adjustment, and occupational status. The effects of only-child status on the homosexual women were explored. Comparisons with other research on female homosexuality and only-child status were made. Fewer homosexuals abstained from alcohol or drank infrequently than did nonhomosexuals. Significantly more homosexuals drank daily. Mothers of homosexuals were more likely than mothers of nonhomosexuals to be frequent drinkers, and mothers of homosexual only children were more often heavier drinkers than were fathers of only children. (Author)

442. Komaridis, K. G. *Lesbians do exist: The myths and realities of working with alcoholic lesbians, a presentation for the non-gay professional.* Paper presented at the National Council on Alcoholism Annual Meeting, Seattle, May 1980.

The author discusses some of her experiences in working with alcoholic lesbians as a counseling psychologist in a rural community in southern Minnesota. Some myths and facts related to working with alcoholic lesbians are presented. Suggestions are offered to the heterosexual woman for dealing with lesbians. (NCALI)

443. Kristi. Lesbians and alcoholism: Part I. *Lesbian Connections,* February 1975, pp. 4–6.

Lesbians are oppressed by straight society, trapped by a subculture that condones drinking, and enslaved by the gay bar, which encourages drinking. The progression from social drinking at a gay bar to alcoholism takes years and begins with just a couple of drinks to relax. Initially, the lesbian alcoholic is seen as a problem drinker. As alcoholism becomes more serious, she may become isolated. Her absence from the community is noticed, as are her loss of control, forgetfulness, and unreliability. Entering into chronic alcoholism she may try to leave the community to join another, start anew, only to fail in her effort to control her drinking. With continued drinking, a vicious cycle is established: desperate drinking to stop the effects of drinking despite the toll taken in physical and mental well-being.

444. Martin, M. Isolation of the lesbian alcoholic. *Frontiers: A Journal of Women's Studies,* 1979, *4,* 32–37.

The author contends that the problems of the lesbian alcoholic include those intrinsic to all women; however, there are also unique needs which arise from the different conditions that contribute to a lesbian's alcoholism. In this article, sociological and psychological factors, specifically isolation, which contribute to alcoholism among lesbians are discussed. Excerpts from the author's journal are provided, including the words and music to a song written by Meg Christian, entitled "For the Alcoholism Center for Women, Los Angeles." (NCALI)

445. O'Donnell, M., Leoffler, V., Pollock, K., & Saunders, Z. *Lesbian health matters.* Santa Cruz, CA: Santa Cruz Women's Health Center, 1980.

An attempt is made by the authors of this booklet to share women's health information in a format that speaks directly to lesbians. Medical and health problems that confront lesbian women are explicitly discussed. In a section entitled "Alcoholism and Co-alcoholism: There is a Solution," it is noted that the alcoholism rate among the gay population is estimated to be more than 3 times that in the general population. The gay bar has been and continues to be a significant part of the homosexual community, and for lesbians, bars provide the only environment where they can be themselves. The following topics are discussed in this section: (1) definitions of alcoholism, (2) how to identify a drinking problem, (3) signs of alcoholism, (4) role and definition of a co-alcoholic, (5) medical and behavioral effects of alcoholism, (6) the effectiveness of recovery programs, and (7) individual and community involvement. (NCALI)

446. Saghir, M. T., Robins, E., Walbran, B., & Gentry, K. A. Homosexuality: IV. Psychiatric disorders and disability in the female homosexual. *American Journal of Psychiatry,* 1970, *127,* 147–154.

A study of 57 homosexual women and 43 single heterosexual controls revealed slightly more clinically significant changes and disability in the lives of homosexual women as compared with the heterosexual women. The chief differences were in prevalence of alcoholism and of attempted suicide. The population was also analyzed on such variables as prevalence of psychiatric disorders in the homosexual female, nonprescription drug use, neuroses and personality disorders, prevalence of psychiatric illness in the parents of female homosexuals, educational and occupational achievement levels, and comparison between psychiatric disorders of females and males. It is concluded that being a homosexual seems to be compatible with functional and interpersonal productivity, although the risk of having a psychiatric disorder and of intrapersonal conflict seems to be greater in the homosexual than in the single heterosexual.

447. Underhill, B. L. *Elements of effective services for the lesbian.* Paper presented at the Third Annual Women in Crisis Conference, New York, June–July 1981.

Some of the essential elements of providing counseling services for the lesbian are outlined, focusing on the cultural factors that make these treatment elements crucial. The following treatment elements are discussed: (1) a supportive and nonjudgmental environment, (2) group therapy, (3) collateral counseling, (4) educational presentations, (5) anger groups, (6) consciousness raising groups, (7) sexuality groups, (8) vocational/skills training, (9) special groups for lesbian mothers who like alcoholic mothers with children face special legal problems, (10) focus on self-esteem, and (11) individualized services. It is noted that for the alcoholic or chemically dependent woman sexuality is a critical issue for treatment and recovery. (NCALI)

448. Weathers, B. *Alcoholism and the lesbian community.* Washington, DC: Gay Council on Drinking Behavior, Whitman-Walker Clinic, 1980.

The high alcoholism rate among lesbians is attributed to 3 factors: (1) the lesbian community constitutes an oppressed minority, (2) the lesbian bar is the traditional setting for social activities, and (3) alcoholism treatment directed toward the needs of the alcoholic lesbian is generally unavailable. Judgmental and restrictive staff attitudes result in negative interactions with alcoholism treatment agencies as follows: (1) refusal of services if lesbianism is known or suspected; (2) service is often provided on a limited basis or in an aversive atmosphere; and (3) services are directed toward lesbianism as the primary problem with little or no attention directed toward alcoholism. Seven points are outlined for improving service delivery and for satisfying the needs of lesbian alcoholics: (1) a safe and nonjudgmental atmosphere, (2) a peer support group, (3) full access to a wide range of services, (4) nontraditional support services, (5) recognition of clients' individuality, (6) increased staff awareness and sensitivity to the lesbian alcoholic, and (7) specialized treatment groups, e.g., lesbian groups, all-women groups, and gay groups for men and women.

3. Males

449. Bell, R. R. Male homosexuality. In R. R. Bell, *Social deviance: A substantive analysis.* Homewood, IL: Dorsey, 1971.

A cross-cultural and historical view is taken in analyzing homosexuality as social deviance. Reviews of the literature on the causes of homosexuality are presented. In the homosexual subculture, the gay bar provides the gathering place for the homosexual community. These bars are discussed in detail, presenting sociological analysis of their growth and function in the community. Within the broader society, homosexuals are beset by legal and social sanctions against their subculture. As public opinion shifts, social changes allow for more comfort on the part of homosexuals. For example, the State Liquor Authority of New York lifted its ban on gay bars, and state courts have ruled that intrasexual touching and dancing are not necessarily disorderly.

450. Daen, P. *The body image and sexual preference of alcoholic, homosexual and heterosexual males.* (Unpublished doctoral dissertation, Adelphi College, 1960).

In a study investigating the relationship between latent homosexuality and alcoholism in males, subjects were asked to indicate preference for male or female pictures presented in paired slide presentations, to indicate preference for pictures of symbols, and to draw a figure. Subjects were 30 homosexuals, 30 alcoholics, and 30 married heterosexuals. The first picture preference test produced significant differences between the 3 groups with the alcoholics falling midway between the other 2 groups in preference. The symbol test did not discriminate between homosexuals and hetero-

sexuals, but ratings of the figure drawings did so discriminate, and as with the picture preference test, alcoholics fell between these 2 groups in the latter. The author concludes that alcoholics have ambiguous sexual orientation and body image.

451. Lohrenz, L. J., Connelly, J. C., Coyne, L., & Spare, K. E. Alcohol problems in several midwestern homosexual communities. *Journal of Studies on Alcohol,* 1978, *39,* 1959–1963.

Data obtained during a questionnaire survey of 145 homosexual men in 4 urban areas in east-central Kansas were analyzed. The 73-item questionnaire included the Michigan Alcoholism Screening Test (MAST) and questions about demographic characteristics, sexual preferences and experiences, use and misuse of alcohol and other drugs, general adjustment, and help-seeking and help-rejecting attitudes. Most of the men surveyed were young (86 were 18–25 and 46 were 26–35); most were from cities (60 from cities of 100,000 or more and 46 from cities of 10,000–100,000); 51 were students, 31 professionals or executives, and 30 were businessmen or craftsmen; all but 18 had attended college. According to MAST scores, 42 (29%) of the men were alcoholics. MAST scores were related to the respondents' perception of alcohol as a solution to problems (p < .001), to residence in a university city or metropolitan setting, to education, to current sexual preference for men, and to perception of prescription drugs as a solution to problems (p < .05). The percentage of homosexual men identified as problem drinkers is similar to that found by L. Fifield, who studied a West Coast population. (RUCAS)

452. Mayo, E. E. The relationship between self-concept variables and sexual preferences among male alcoholics and male non-alcoholics (Doctoral dissertation, University of Colorado at Boulder, 1979). *Dissertation Abstracts International,* 1980, *40,* 4413B. (University Microfilms No. 80-02,997)

The purpose of this study was to determine if significant differences existed in self-concept based on sexual preference and alcoholism. To test hypotheses of this study, 120 males between 20 and 35 years of age and employed were divided into 4 groups based on their identified sexual preference and alcoholic status. The groups were: (1) alcoholic homosexuals, (2) alcoholic heterosexuals, (3) homosexual nonalcoholics, and (4) heterosexual nonalcoholics. The groups were compared to each other on the Total P Score and on the remaining 28 variables from the Tennessee Self-concept Scale. The results of the study indicate that significant differences in self-concept as identified by the Total P Score exist between homosexual alcoholics and homosexual nonalcoholics, homosexual alcoholics and heterosexual nonalcoholics, heterosexual alcoholics and homosexual nonalcoholics, and heterosexual alcoholics and heterosexual nonalcoholics. No significant differences were found in the Total P Score between homosexual nonalcoholics and heterosexual nonalcoholics, or between homosexual alcoholics and heterosexual alcoholics. (Author)

453. Polo, C. A. *Common sense approach to working with gay alcoholics.* Paper presented at the meeting of the Alcohol and Drug Problem Association, New Orleans, 1976.

The alcoholism counselor should consider alcohol, not sexual preference, to be the male gay alcoholic's primary problem. Alcohol is chosen as a means of coping with social tensions related to the gay lifestyle. There are 5 factors that influence gays' behavior and that need to be considered in the counselling: (1) subgroup membership (e.g., leather or S & M), (2) source of social contacts, (3) living and relationship arrangements, (4) family acceptance, and (5) closed or open affirmation of sexuality. The paper discusses these 5 factors in detail. The gay man who is stigmatized as an alcoholic loses his desirability, a problem for the polygamous gay. He is rejected by his peers and left to the role of sexual isolate. The recovering gay alcoholic must realize that his previous source of sexual and social contact may no longer be appropriate or conducive to continuous sobriety. The counselor must be able to acquaint him with alternative sources. Both gay and nongay A.A. groups can provide social alternatives.

454. Saghir, M. T., Robins, E., Walbran, B., & Gentry, K. A. Homosexuality: III. Psychiatric disorders and disability in the male homosexual. *American Journal of Psychiatry*, 1970, *126*, 1079–1086.

Information concerning clinical psychiatric illness among male homosexuals is presented. Based on an interview technique, little difference was demonstrated in the prevalence of psychopathology between a group of 89 male homosexuals and a control group of 35 unmarried heterosexual men. When differences did occur they were in the direction of more difficulties among the homosexual subjects than among the heterosexual controls. The increased difficulties for the homosexual subjects included a slightly higher prevalence of manifest psychopathology and difficulty in coping with it. Affective disorders, excessive drinking, disability related to psychiatric illness, and attempted suicide were more common among the homosexual group. It is concluded that despite these differences the homosexual subjects were able to achieve educational, occupational, and economic status similar to that of controls.

455. Small, E. J., Jr., & Leach, B. Counseling homosexual alcoholics: Ten case histories. *Journal of Studies on Alcohol*, 1977, *38*, 2077–2086.

The case histories of 10 male homosexual alcoholics are presented, and psychoanalytic theories about the link between homosexuality and alcoholism are reviewed. These case histories are believed to typify the coincidental occurrence of alcoholism and homosexuality in men in contemporary American culture. They appear to illustrate the hypothesis that the 2 conditions are likely to coexist circumstantially rather than causatively. None of the patients discussed fits the stereotype of the male homosexual. Their personality types vary widely, as do their homosexual activities and drinking behaviors. The traditional view that homosexuality causes alcoholism may be erroneous, even antitherapeutic. Recovery from pathological drinking seemed to be within reach almost as soon as the patient could view alcoholism as a condition independent of homosexuality. These homosexual alcoholics responded to treatment for alcoholism when the therapy did not demand they become heterosexual.

456. Smith, T. M. *Specific approaches and techniques in the treatment of gay male alcohol abusers.* San Francisco, CA: Department of Public Health, Alcoholism Evaluation and Treatment Center, 1979.

In this report, it is noted that available statistics indicate that approximately one-third of gay male adults in cosmopolitan areas are alcohol abusers, and that one gay male in 10 in the general population is an alcohol abuser. General treatment approach principles both for gay clients and "alcoholics" are discussed. In ths paper, the bias of treatment approaches is toward individualized, interpersonal, holistic eclecticism: a combination of responsibility building therapy, awareness therapy, medical and neurophysiological approaches, strategic therapy, utilization of altered states of consciousness, and attitudinal change therapy. A highlighted discussion of specific therapeutic techniques and approaches to the "gay male alcoholic" is also presented. (RUCAS)

457. Smith, T. M. *Factors involved in individualizing strategic psychotherapy and holistic approaches to the treatment of gay male alcohol abusers.* San Francisco, CA: Department of Public Health, Alcoholism Evaluation and Treatment Center, 1980.

The report discusses strategic and holistic therapeutic approaches which incorporate an appreciation of the gay male alcoholic, both as a gay individual and as a person involved in a biophysical disorder. The following factors are delineated: (1) client's attitudes and value systems, (2) client's participation in the general society and in the gay subculture, (3) gay milieus, (4) the protean nature of sexuality, (5) life strategies of gay men, (6) the "coming out" process, (7) gay language and sensibilities, and (8) compound symptoms, i.e., symptoms shared in common by alcoholism and the oppression of gay people. Brief case material is presented, describing how each of these factors is utilized to individualize treatment for gay male alcohol abusers. (RUCAS)

458. Turner, W. J. Alcoholism, homosexuality, and bipolar affective disorder. *American Journal of Psychiatry*, 1981, *138*, 262–263.

In view of the relatively frequent occurrence of bipolar affective disorder, homosexuality, and alcoholism in the same family and the evidence that depression or alcoholism frequently accompanies homosexuality, the possibility that some male homosexuality is genetically determined as part of a familial common disorder warrants investigation. (RUCAS)

459. Weinberg, M. S., & Williams, C. J. *Male homosexuals.* New York: Oxford University Press, 1974.

The results of sociological field work that began in 1966 are presented in this book. Questionnaires were distributed at gay bars, at functions held by homophile societies, and through mailings. Data were collected from 1,057 American homosexuals (in New York, Connecticut, New Jersey, and the San Francisco area), 1,077 homosexuals in the Netherlands, and 303 Danish homosexuals. The focus of the study was to examine the influence of demographic and social factors on adjustment to homosexual life. The function of the gay bar is discussed for its importance as a meeting place for socializing and establishing sexual contacts.

460. Ziebold, T. O., & Mongeon, J. E. *Treatment strategies for homosexual alcoholics in recovery and reconstruction.* Paper presented at the National Council on Alcoholism Annual Meeting, Seattle, May 1980.

It is the authors' observation that gay alcoholics at the outset of recovery are fearful and uncertain as to how they relate not only to the heterosexual world but also to the homosexual community. Selected topics to be considered in the treatment of gay alcoholics both in early recovery (initial abstinence) and in the phase of recovery entered after one to 2 years of sobriety (reconstruction) are discussed. The discussion is limited to a certain population, i.e., gay men in an urban social setting. The following 4 aspects of the reality of being homosexual which alcoholics do not manage well are discussed: (1) living in a hostile society, (2) having the option of "passing" for heterosexual, (3) fulfilling homosexually oriented intimacy needs, and (4) feeling worthwhile without the benefit of meeting society's expectations of being spouses or parents. Specific recommendations for addressing these aspects are offered. (NCALI)

461. Ziebold, T. O., & Mongeon, J. E. *Ways to gay sobriety.* Washington, DC: Gay Council on Drinking Behavior, Whitman-Walker Clinic, 1980.

This pamphlet is the printed version of a presentation to the National Council on Alcoholism annual meeting in Seattle, May 1980. The authors report their observation that gay alcoholics at the beginning of sobriety are fearful and uncertain. The newly sober gay alcoholic has little experience relating to other gays except as a sex object and has little experience surviving in an often hostile society without alcohol and compulsive sex as means of escape. The task in early sobriety for gays, as for other alcoholics, is to get over the focus on alcohol in social interaction and the compulsion to use alcohol in dealing with stress. Once comfortable with abstinence, the gay alcoholic is faced with the task of reconstructing a gay life without alcohol, a task which all too often is made more difficult by the lack of social support and successful gay role models. Prominent issues for homosexual alcoholics are: (1) living in a hostile society, (2) the option of "passing" for heterosexual, (3) differentiating homosexual intimacy from lust and learning to fulfill intimacy needs, and (4) maintaining self-esteem while living outside of societal expectations. The authors recommend treatment planning which includes: (1) emphasis on development of intimacy and exploration of nonsexual physical contact, (2) encouraging activities that are esteem enhancing for gays, such as attending to physical attractiveness and participating in playful sexual encounters, (3) focus on the emotional loss process and necessity for reaching out to others, (4) exercises to help deal with anger, and (5) focus on positive aspects of gay identity. (NCALI)

D. Cross-cultural and Historical Reports

462. Bishop, G. Sex. In G. Bishop, *The booze reader*. Los Angeles, CA: Sherbourne Press, 1965.

The longstanding association between sex and alcohol is illustrated with historical anecdotes reaching as far back as ancient China. Reflecting on these, as well as on modern day occurrences involving alcohol and sex, the author concludes that the setting in which the alcohol is imbibed, not the alcohol, determines a person's conduct with regard to sexuality.

463. Boyer, L. B. Psychological problems of a group of Apaches: Alcoholic hallucinosis and latent homosexuality among typical men. In W. Muensterberger & S. Axelrad (Eds.), *The psychoanalytic study of society* (Vol. 3). New York: International Universities Press, 1964.

In this anthropological study of reservation-bound Apaches, personality development, social structure, and the socialization process are examined from a psychoanalytic perspective. Alcoholic hallucinosis is a serious problem among the Apache and psychotic episodes are attributed to ghosts and witches. Aggressive and promiscuous behavior is common, overt, and tolerated. While the behaviors may be unacceptable, drunkenness excuses individuals from responsibility for their actions. Overt homosexuality is nearly unheard of, which represents a massive denial embedded in the Apache cultural heritage. Children are raised with ambivalent contradictory values and mores and are exposed to repeated exhibitions of sexual activity and brutality perpetrated by intoxicated adults. As a result, adult sexual identity is inadequate. Drunkenness is used as a culturally approved outlet for poorly integrated sexual and aggressive energies.

464. Branson, H. *Gay bar*. San Francisco, CA: Pan Graphic, 1957.

The use of alcohol by homosexuals in a bar setting is discussed. Specific emphasis is placed on the physiological and psychological functions of alcohol in the homosexual subculture.

465. Bunzel, R. The role of alcoholism in two Central American cultures. *Psychiatry*, 1940, *3*, 361–387.

Residents in 2 villages were studied: Chichicastenango in Guatemala and Chamula in Mexico. In Chichicastenango alcohol is consumed on market days and at festivals. More men than women drink. Zarabandas, dancing parties at which alcohol is sold, are held several times a year. On these occasions promiscuous, erotic behavior is common, in sharp contrast with the extreme decorum observed at other times and in conflict with the culture's strict rules on sexual morality. Drinking is associated with quarrels and sexual license, violation of the 2 basic rules of domestic life. Drunkenness is feared for the disruptions that follow drunken behavior. In Chamula everyone drinks, including children, who are introduced to alcohol in early infancy. Drinking is done in groups and is a part of every ceremonial and social contact, yet there is a notable absence of erotic behavior accompanying drinking.

466. Devereux, G. The function of alcohol in Mohave society. *Quarterly Journal of Studies on Alcohol*, 1948, *9*, 207–251.

Alcohol is used for sexual purposes in quite a different way from its use by Whites since sexual relations are not considered vile or antisocial by the Mohave; an offer of a drink by a man to a woman and her acceptance of it is an implicit offer and consent to sexual intercourse. Since the main sexual stimulus is simply opportunity, alcohol fits into this pattern; the woman invited to go on a spree (alcoholic and, implicitly, sexual) may be the man's own wife; a woman who becomes intoxicated knows that she will surely be raped by one or more men around her (which may include her husband). Maudlin sentimentality is lacking among the Mohave when they drink. They seem to behave as they always do, "only more so." Since they are able to express their feelings freely, they do not need to get drunk to do so nor do they indulge in outbursts of sadism. The Mohave do not need to purchase courage and social approval through self-inflicted suffering in an essentially hostile world. The intoxicated Mohave is not usually aggressive, and drunken brawls are rare. This phenomenon is analyzed from various viewpoints, and explanations are sought. The stoic courage of the Mohave is a living force among them, and no man is compelled to validate his claims for bravery; their ideal is a man who combines gentleness with stoic courage. In aboriginal times aggressions were expressed in war with neighbors; after the White occupation the Mohave found a new and to them acceptable "alternate" behavior: they became sex-specialists. Illustrative examples are cited of Mohave behavior under alcohol and their attitude to drinking and drunkenness. (RUCAS)

467. Devereaux, G. The function of alcohol. In G. Deveraux, *Mohave ethnopsychiatry and suicide: The psychiatric knowledge and the psychic disturbances of an Indian tribe*. St. Clair Shores, MI: Scholarly Press,

1976. (Smithsonian Institution Bureau of American Ethnology Bulletin 175. Originally published, Washington, DC: U.S. Government Printing Office, 1961.)

Alcohol came to play an important role in Mohave life in the late 1800s when disreputable Whites, moving westward, used alcohol for economic and sexual exploitation of Indians. Indian women were lured into prostitution to obtain alcohol, and the workmen's camps surrounding construction projects provided the marketplace. Mohave drinking is typically moderate and done in a social setting, e.g., in a gathering of friends, at a dance, or at a party. The Mohave strongly condemn excessive drinking. Alcoholism is associated with witchcraft and incest in Mohave culture. Moderate drinking, as long as it does not lead to sex orgies or aggressive behavior, is considered normal and pleasurable. Drinking in connection with sex is distinguished from hospitality drinking. An unattached man will share his alcohol with a woman with whom he wishes to have intercourse or with a group of adventurous men and women. Acceptance is implicit consent to engage in sex. However, alcohol is rarely used for seduction or payment for sexual favors. Alcohol intoxication is seen as an opportunity for sex. A woman who becomes intoxicated is aware that her state constitutes an invitation to the men in the group to "take turns on her." Promiscuous alcoholic women are severely abused sexually in punitive mass rapes and genital mutilation. Psychoanalytic interpretations of Mohave behavior reveal the Mohave to have achieved, as a culture, a reasonably high degree of psychosexual maturity.

468. Erdoes, R. "Wimmin," or only a bird in a gilded cage, or women, good and bad. In R. Erdoes, *Saloons of the Old West*. New York: Alfred A. Knopf, 1979.

The saloons of the old West catered to the frontiersman's strongest appetites. The miners and cowboys went to saloons to drink with hope of finding "sportin' women" who would drink with them and entertain them. Women were scarce in the old West, and those who ventured to the mining towns and cattle towns easily found employment at local saloons. They worked as "pretty waiter girls," serving customers in costumes that ranged from a country girl's Sunday dress to nothing but a jacket and plumed bonnet, or they may have been "hurdy gals" whose occupation was to dance with the customers and encourage customers to buy them drinks. Saloons of this type were the hurdy-gurdy houses or honkytonks. Hurdy gals and waiter girls led unconventional lives, taking lovers freely, but they were seldom prostitutes. Some became wives and mothers, elevating themselves to status of "good women." Prostitutes could most reliably be found in "dancing saloons." Women sang and danced on stage, mingled with the customers to encourage them to buy drinks, and sold sexual favors in upstairs rooms, back rooms, or curtained private areas. At first, "good women" tolerated the presence of prostitutes and honky-tonkers, seeing them as protection from the unwanted advances from the drunken men who came out of the wilderness with "squaw fever." In later years, as the numbers of women in the West grew, "fancy women" were no longer seen as protection but as competition. Good women began lending support to Eastern preachers who condemned the dance halls and saloons. Legislation prohibiting employment of women to attract and entertain customers was passed throughout the West, successfully closing down saloons, dance halls, and hurdy-gurdy houses.

469. Hamer, J., & Steinbring, J. *Alcohol and native peoples of the North*. Lanham, MD: University Press of America, 1980.

Patterns of drinking behavior in relationship to a variety of social behaviors, including sex, are explored for their meaning in North American Indian cultures. In light of contemporary North American Indian drinking practices and their historical antecedents, the hypothesis is advanced that "the amount of drinking and drunken comportment varies with the extent to which Native people are able to establish satisfying individual and group identity, succeed by their own assertiveness to desirable positions, and achieve a balance between the expression of self-reliance and dependency within and between ethnic groups." It is concluded that the prognosis for any attempt to "improve" these drinking customs is exceedingly poor. (RUCAS)

470. Hill, T. W. Life styles and drinking patterns of urban Indians. *Journal of Drug Issues*, 1980, *10*, 257–272.

Lifestyles and drinking patterns of the Winnebago and Santee Dakota Indians of Sioux City, IA, were studied by interviews, analysis of agency records and written documents, and by extensive participant observation during a 12-month period in 1970–1971. Drinking activities were seen in terms of the Indians' cultural systems. A dyadic discrimination test and several card-sorting tasks, in addition to interviewing and observation, showed that study participants distinguished 7 types of people: somebodies (professionals), everyday people, people who like to raise hell, individuals who don't think of trouble, family men, people on the street, and periodic "drunks." In contrast to researchers who argue that a single set of drinking standards or norms is shared across ethnic and class lines in the U.S., it is shown that the Indians of Sioux City use multiple sets of drinking patterns and that some sets define some forms of heavy and frequent drinking as acceptable behavior. The majority of respondents considered the range of acceptable drinking to lie between the 2 extremes of total abstinence and nearly continuous intoxication. The specific standard for a given individual within a particular relationship and situation is usually based on decisions reached through social interaction. The "people who like to raise hell" are the heaviest drinkers. This group strives toward asserting masculine prowess in their drinking, premarital sex, and illegal activities. With age, "hell raisers" settle down, marry, and become "family men." Sexual and illegal exploits are put aside, and drinking is diminished. Unsuccessful transition from "hell raiser" to "family man" results in joining "people on the street" or the "drunks." (RUCAS)

471. Hippler, A. E. Patterns of sexual behavior: The Athabascans of interior Alaska. *Ethos*, 1974, *2*, 47–68.

There is a strong tendency toward orgiastic sex and violence, misuse of alcohol, and antisocial sexual activity for the

Athabascans. Strong antagonism between the males and females is acted out in the sexual arena in patterns of avoidance, teasing, and violent sexual encounters. Sex itself is viewed as evil and dirty, and strong cultural restraints against sexual activity exist. Sexual activity is usually delayed until around age 20, occurring in the teens only in families lacking adult controls. Girls begin in early puberty to develop and refine skills involved in sexuality by teasing older men who are drunk, then running away before actual sexual contact is made. Drinking is often the prelude to sex, and presence of a woman at a drinking party leads to tension. If she becomes intoxicated, it is taken as a signal of sexual intentions. Violence due to jealousy and/or rape are common outcomes. Among many married couples, the husband signals his intention for intercourse by becoming intoxicated and beating his wife. The Athabascans have a cultural heritage of restrictive sexual expression. Contact with Whites has lead to the breakdown of their highly structured society resulting in alcohol excesses and explosive sexual behavior.

472. Honigmann, J. J., & Honigmann, I. Drinking in an Indian-white community. *Quarterly Journal of Studies on Alcohol,* 1945, *5,* 575–619.

During the summer of 1944, the authors lived as members of a small trading post in Northern Canada. Behavior related to the acquisition and consumption of alcohol was recorded as was behavior during and following intoxication. The Indians, who were legally forbidden to drink alcoholic beverages, secretly brewed malt beer. Alcohol appeared to facilitate social interaction, release sexual inhibition, and release inhibitions concerning aggression. The White men drank commercial as well as home-brewed beverages. White women were never observed drinking. Drunken behavior of the White men was manifested in uninhibited friendliness to each other, reckless behavior, practical jokes, and clowning. Sexual desire was heightened. Some men used alcohol to win access to Indian women; others told obscene jokes. In contrast to the Indians, alcohol did not have a marked disinhibiting effect on sexual or aggressive behavior among Whites. Since there were only 21 Whites, fighting would increase the Whites' isolation. The fact that Whites tended to be older, (average age 45), and when sober were not as inhibited sexually as the Indians, may account for the differences in sexual behavior when intoxicated.

473. Horton, D. The functions of alcohol in primitive societies: A cross-cultural study. *Quarterly Journal of Studies on Alcohol,* 1943, *4,* 199–320.

The psychological and physiological effects of alcohol are reviewed. The relationship of inhibition and anxiety and the effects of alcohol on them are explained. Data on 56 societies (12 Asian, 13 African, 6 Oceanic, 11 North American, and 14 South American) from the files of the Cross-Cultural Survey in the Institute of Human Relations, Yale University, were analyzed with respect to use of alcoholic beverages. Release of sexual responses during drinking festivities was reported in 11 societies. Subsistence insecurity was significantly correlated with greater male insobriety. Excluding societies with high subsistence insecurity, a negative association was found between premarital sexual freedom and insobriety. Three patterns emerged: in societies with high subsistence anxiety and strong belief in sorcery, insobriety was always excessive and accompanied by extreme aggression; societies with high subsistence anxiety without belief in sorcery showed excessive insobriety with moderate aggression; the third pattern was fear and restraint in drinking. A table presents a list of societies and ratings on 10 characteristics: degree of insobriety, type of economy, subsistence insecurity, frequency of warfare with respect to economy and to warfare, acculturation, sorcery, premarital restraint, type of beverage available, and alcoholic aggression.

474. Kuttner, R. E. Poverty and sex: Relationships in a "skid row" slum. *Sexual Behavior,* 1971, *1,* 55–63.

This study investigated Indian and Appalachian groups in a skid row in the Uptown district of Chicago. Alcoholism, petty crime, unemployment, promiscuity, and lack of skills were identified as contributors to the demoralization of the people. Findings were consistent with the accepted opinion that sexual activity in skid row areas is simplified, mechanistic, and essentially unromantic. However, the author concludes that the difference between skid row and middle-class women is not in standards, but in success in adhering to standards. Such success may be attributed as much to social circumstances as to inherited qualities.

475. Levine, S. Crime or affliction? Rape in an African community. *Culture Medicine and Psychiatry,* 1980, *4,* 151–165.

A case is presented of a teacher of the Gusii of southwestern Kenya, who was fired because of alcoholism. However, his problem was not only alcoholism, as indicated by his sexual attacks on a number of women and young girls and his attempted rape of a teenage niece. Since boyhood, he had infringed the rules of kin–avoidance between generations. His abhorrent behavior occurred when he was drunk, that is, in a transitional state in which ipso facto he was not responsible for his actions. In Guisiiland, alcohol commonly allows for the violent acting out of paranoid fantasies, and people who are generally congenial are allowed, when drunk, to behave in a way from which they disassociate themselves entirely when sober. (RUCAS)

476. Matthiasson, J. S. You scratch my back and I'll scratch yours: Continuities in Inuit social relationships. In J. Hamer & J. Steinbring (Eds.), *Alcohol and native peoples of the North.* Lanham, MD: University Press of America, 1980.

The avoidance of drinking-related interpersonal violence among the Inuit of northern Baffin Island is described. Social networks among Inuit men are maintained by drinking, and the traditional avoidance of socially damaging expressions of interpersonal hostility prevents violence. It is suggested that drinking among the Inuit is not as socially and psychologically disruptive as some casual observers have concluded. (RUCAS)

477. McClelland, D. C., Davis, W. N., Wanner, E., & Kalin, R. A cross-cultural study of folk-tale content and drinking. *Sociometry,* 1966, *29,* 308–333.

A representative sample of independent cultures was carefully chosen to check cross-cultural correlates of drinking and the folktale themes associated with it. Analysis of the folktales was carried out by the computer-based General Inquirer System, which coded the content according to some 88 tags of which 14 tags yielded significant correlations with drinking. As in previous studies, several societal variables (such as hunting and indices of simple social structure) were correlated with drinking, but the associated folktale theme suggests that the psychological state involved is not subsistence anxiety or need for dependence as previous authors have argued, but a feeling of weakness in the face of heavy demands, which leads men to dream of magical potency and to seek it by heavy drinking. Sober societies provide more structural support for the individual and instill the virtues of respect and activity inhibition that suit such a society and control drinking. Sexual themes correlated with drinking and several subtypes of sexual imagery (affiliative, male-dominated, female-dominated, male rivalry) varied in the size of correlations with drinking from one sample to another. (Author)

478. Norick, F. A. Acculturation and drinking in Alaska. *Rehabilitation Record*, 1970, *11*, 13–17.

This article is an exerpt from a report by Dr. Norick on a study of acculturation and social maladjustment among the native peoples of Alaska. The widespread and indiscriminate use of alcoholic beverages among Alaska's native peoples is a problem that is generally thought to be of the greatest concern. It is almost always associated there with a wide range of other deviant actions, including job instability, sexual promiscuity, and minor transgressions against society, e.g., petty theft, disorderly conduct, and similar misdemeanors. The possibility of obtaining sexual gratification is often regarded as a natural adjunct to drinking parties, and sex is often responsible for outbreaks of hostility, particularly if the party is attended by White males. Apart from its convivial function, alcohol serves as a medicine for the ills and misfortunes of the aged. Occasionally, older women, especially widows, will purchase liquor which serves to secure the company of older men.

479. O'Carroll, M. D. The relationship of religion and ethnicity to drinking behavior: A study of North European immigrants in the United States (Doctoral dissertation, University of California, Berkeley, 1979). *Dissertation Abstracts International*, 1980, *40*, 4236B. (University Microfilms No. 80-00,256)

The relative effects of religion and ethnicity on the drinking behavior and drinking practices of Irish Catholics in the United States was studied, and the validity of previous sociological theories regarding Irish Catholic drinking practices was tested, as was a novel theory that associates Irish Catholic drinking practices and problems with a relatively tolerant religious normative structure. The novel theoretical model posits that the conflict caused by the relationship of an authoritarian religious institution and its psychologically dependent constituency initiates a routinized cycle of rebellion (abusive drinking) and resentment (confession, forgiveness, and reincorporation into group life) that is easily transferrable from religious to secular domains. It is hypothesized that it is functionally imperative for Catholic ecclesiastics both to maintain institutional authority and to enforce prohibitive norms surrounding premarital sex, by concurrently tolerating deviant drinking practices and generally permitting a lax normative regulation of alcohol consumption by its constituents in order to discharge psychosexual tension in the relationship. This novel theoretical orientation was initially specified in 6 hypothetical associations of the psychosocial and institutional elements previously described (ecclesial authority, drinking practices, religious affiliation, ethnic identity, and attitudes toward alcohol consumption), and a series of quantitative tests of these hypothesized relationships was initiated by rigorously analyzing survey reseach data integrated from 6 separate national community studies conducted in 1959–1964. (RUCAS)

480. Quaife, G. R. The consenting spinster in a peasant society: Aspects of premarital sex in "puritan" Somerset 1645–1660. *Journal of Social History*, 1977, *11*, 228–244.

This is a study of sexual behavior among the working people of Somerset, England in the mid-1600s. The study made use of parish records, records from ecclesiastical courts, and records from justices of the peace concerned with bastardy jurisdiction. Records of the Quarter Sessions and the information, depositions, and examinations contained in the Session Rolls provide descriptions of sexual behavior and the circumstances under which premarital intercourse took place. Most incidents of premarital intercourse took place under promise by the male to marry the consenting female. Peaks in sexual activity occurred during festival seasons when eating, heavy drinking, and sex were part of the festivities. Unmarried females rarely went to inns or "tippling houses." These were the haunts of wanton widows and wayward wives. Young females entering an inn would be mistaken for whores. Young women who did frequent drinking places and drank with disreputable company were few. They were likely to be abused and their fate considered a just reward for their behavior. Drinking alcohol was commonly practiced by all. Every man, woman, and child consumed over a pint of beer daily. Young, unmarried women organized their own drinking parties, an acceptable practice at the time. Depositions describing the circumstances of a seduction commonly include alcohol. Men were reported to encourage unmarried girls to drink to make them more willing to consent to intercourse.

481. Roebuck, J., & Spray, S. L. The cocktail lounge: A study of heterosexual relations in a public organization. *American Journal of Sociology*, 1967, *72*, 388–395.

This paper covers a body of data in a relatively neglected area of research, namely, the social life found in a high-status public organization. Using a variety of methods (participant observation, interviews, having the employees of the organization systematically gather data on the clientele), it was found that the cocktail lounge was frequented by regular patrons who engaged in organized activities around which stable expectations for "proper" behavior had developed. The major function of the cocktail lounge was the facilitation of casual sexual affairs between high-status married men and young, unattached women. The organization of the cocktail lounge is described, and the relationship between activities in the lounge and outside social ties is discussed. (Author)

482. Salonen, A. Dryckesseder före och efter Muhammed. [Drinking customs before and after Mohammed.] *Alkoholpolitik,* 1958, *21,* 50–52.

Mohammed contributed to more restrained consumption of alcoholic beverages in Arabic countries through his writings and the example of his own behavior. Information on drinking customs was gathered from poetry, from the Koran and other religious writings, and from traditional lore. Earliest Arabic poetry depicts Jewish and Christian wine merchants, nomads who bought their ''wine shop'' tents to Bedouin camps. The merchants always employed beautiful females to entertain customers with music and orgies. Under the influence of Mohammed, Arabic customs returned to more restrictive behaviors, which had their roots in the ancient Semitic idea that in wine and music lurks a demon.

E. Alcohol and Sexuality in the Media

483. Beckley, R. E., & Chalfant, H. P. Contrasting images of alcohol and drug use in country and rock music. *Journal of Alcohol and Drug Education*, 1979, *25*, 44–51.

The texts of 275 country and 250 rock songs chosen in 1974–1975 from *Billboard* magazine's lists of top 100 favorites songs were examined for thier concern with alcohol and drug use and abuse. Whereas 39 of the 42 rock music songs with drug content reflected no ambivalence toward drug use (all but 2 portrayed it as desirable or normal), 25 of the 30 country music songs that mentioned alcohol reflected ambivalence over the use of alcoholic beverages. All 30 country country songs suggested some values concerning drinking, and in all but 7 both the ideal of alcohol as evil and its real value as an expected part of living were expressed. Only 7 of these 30 songs failed to indicate either facilitating behavior or assuaging problem (loneliness, failure, guilt) as reasons for drinking. (RUCAS)

484. Blair, E., Sudman, S., Bradburn, N. M., & Stocking, C. How to ask questions about drinking and sex: Response effects in measuring consumer behavior. *Journal of Marketing Research*, 1977, *14*, 316–321.

This article reports a nationwide study of response effects based on answers from almost 1,200 respondents to threatening behavioral questions presented in various formats. Results indicated that threatening questions requiring yes-or-no answers can be asked in any format, but that threatening questions requiring quantified answers are best asked in open-ended, long questions with respondent-familiar wording. (Author)

485. Breed, W., & De Foe, J. R. Themes in magazine alcohol advertisements: A critique. *Journal of Drug Issues*, 1979, *9*, 511–522.

From a sample of 13 widely circulated national magazines, including those predominantly used by men, women, and minority groups, 454 alcohol advertisements were analyzed. Most prominent were advertisements with indirect appeals associating the beverage with a desired outcome state—frequently a lifestyle. In order of frequency, the themes featured wealth-prestige-success, social approval, relaxation-leisure, hedonistic pleasure, exotic associations, individualistic behavior, and sexuality. The relationship between these values and the beverage was absent. Other appeals—direct, covert, and history-tradition-heritage—were also found. The advertisements were basically unrealistic and rested heavily on fantasy. A conceptual scheme for understanding the phenomenon is presented, and several questions are posed for future policy consideration by the government and the alcohol industry. (Author)

486. Cook, J., & Lewington, M. (Eds.). *Images of alcoholism*. London: British Film Institute, 1979.

The essays in this book are revisions of papers given at a conference on 'The Representation of Alcoholism in Cinema and Television'' held at the National Film Theatre (England) in September 1978. General considerations include the portrayal of alcoholism treatment and stereotypes of alcoholics in the movies, women and alcohol, the alcoholic as a hero, and drinking on television. It is suggested that much of the drinking behavior portrayed as harm-free drinking is very harmful from the clinical point of view, and that the films do not adequately deal with the area of alcohol-produced physical damage.

487. Marsteller, P., & Karnchanapee, K. The use of women in the advertising of distilled spirits 1956–1979. *Journal of Psychedelic Drugs*, 1980, *12*, 1–12.

Images of women in distilled spirits advertising before and after the ban against it was lifted on November 20, 1958 are compared. Reproductions of advertisements from mass circulation magazines such as the *New Yorker* illustrate that, despite guidelines from government and industry, the advertising agencies have succeeded in associating romance, glamour, and sexual success with drinking—be it wine, beer, or distilled spirits. It appears that advertisers do not follow the 1975 recommendations of the National Advertising Review Board on avoiding sexual stereotypes, double entendre, and the promise of unrealistic psychological rewards for using the product. (RUCAS)

488. Mosher, J. F., & Wallack, L. M. Proposed reforms in the regulation of alcoholic beverage advertising. *Contemporary Drug Problems*, Spring 1979, 87–106.

It is proposed that alcoholic beverage advertising is misleading in 2 ways: (1) beverages are promoted by appeals to desires and needs that are irrelevant to the product, and (2) the absence of accurate health information in the marketing hampers the consumer's informed choice. The Bureau of Alcohol, Tobacco, and Firearms should use its authority to regulate alcoholic beverage advertising and to ensure that ''irrelevant'' matters likely to mislead consumers by conveying an overall inaccurate impression are not used. Accurate information on social and health problems associated with the use of alcoholic beverages should be transmitted as frequently and with the same intensity as appeals to consumers to buy these products. Ideally, health information should be provided in all alcoholic advertisements. (RUCAS)

IV. Literature Review and Commentary Articles

Introduction

Introduction

A substantial number of articles on alcohol and sexuality cut across several of the categories employed in the first 3 chapters of this bibliography. Many are efforts to integrate several facets of sexual behavior to form a holistic image of the relationship between sex and alcohol. These have been placed in this final chapter and divided into 3 sections.

Section A consists of broadly based literature reviews on sex and alcohol. These reviews extend beyond the domain of any one section of the previous 3 chapters. Literature reviews on more specific topics can be found elsewhere in the appropriate section.

Section B presents representative publications from the psychoanalytic literature. Many of these are early theoretical formulations dating back to the beginning of this century. The publications abstracted here provide psychoanalytic interpretations of alcohol-related phenomena such as delirious behavior during alcoholic psychosis and fantasies during hangover. They also argue that latent homosexuality is an underlying cause of alcoholism.

Section C gathers together all non-data-based publications offering commentary on topics too broad to fit into specific categories. These include proceedings of conferences, interviews, panel discussions, and workshop proceedings. Nonpsychoanalytic theoretical speculations relating to sex and alcohol can be found here along with summaries of information on sex, alcohol, and alcoholism which are not genuine literature reviews.

A. Literature Review

489. Abel, E. L. A review of alcohol's effects on sex and reproduction. *Drug and Alcohol Dependence*, 1980, *5*, 321–332.

The author concludes from his review of the literature that alcohol increases libido, inhibits sexual physiological responses, and adversely affects reproductive processes in men and women. Both men and women report that they feel sexually aroused when under the influence of alcohol, and both experience sexual dysfunction when inebriated. However, alcohol has a greater impact upon male reproductive processes by virtue of the need to achieve and maintain penile vaginal entry and ejaculatory capability. As a result, the probability of a male alcoholic inseminating a female is diminished. In the case of the female, however, the increased sexual arousal stimulated by alcohol will have the effect of increasing the probability of insemination, especially in the case of the female alcoholic, if indeed she is more likely to be promiscuous. Alcohol adversely affects both male and female reproductive physiology. Alcohol not only reduces male hormone production, it also affects spermatogenesis, resulting in the possibility of a male alcoholic siring a defective child. Alcohol also affects female reproductive physiology resulting in increased infertility and an increased likelihood of damage to a developing fetus.

490. Barrucand, D. Alcool et sexualité. [Alcohol and sexuality.] *Alcool ou Sante*, 1980, *152*, 41–44.

Clinical observations of and experimental research on the role of alcohol in sexual excitation of nonalcoholic and alcoholic male and female subjects are reported. In most nonalcoholic subjects, alcohol acts as a stimulant of sexual activity. In alcoholic subjects, alcohol promotes the desire but diminishes quality of sexual experience. Frequent sexual deviations, incest, rape, and homosexuality are correlated with alcoholism. In both normal and alcoholic subjects, alcohol decreases testosterone and luteinizing hormone (LH) levels. Impotence and homosexuality in alcoholics are interpreted in terms of modern psychoanalytical theory. (NCALI)

491. Barrucand, D. Alcool et sexualité. [Alcohol and sexuality.] *Revue de l'Alcoolisme*, 1980, *26*, 71–82.

492. Bruno, F., & Ferracuti, F. Droga e condotte sessuali. [Drugs and sexual behavior.] *Quaderni Criminologia Clinica*, 1977, *19*, 17–36.

Literature on the effects of drugs, including alcohol, on sexual drive and behavior is reviewed. The scientific litera-ture on the addictions and alcoholism does not include many papers on the subject of sexual behaviors under the effect of self-administration of drugs. The results of the studies and of the experiments carried out in this field do not allow a classification of drugs in homogeneous groups according to their specific actions on sexual behavior. For each of the most common drugs the most reliable existing data have been examined. Final conclusions cannot be reached for each drug, since several substances may often act, according to many variables, in different cases as depressants or stimulants. The need to study this aspect of drug addiction and alcoholism has been underlined with the aim to improve our knowledge both in the field of the new sexual therapies and of the prevention and control of drug addiction. (English abstract and English title were provided as a summary at the end of foreign article cited above.) (Author)

493. Langone, J., & Langone, D. D. *Women who drink*. Reading, MA: Addison-Wesley, 1980.

This book about alcoholic women includes discussions on the characteristics of alcoholic women and the etiology, complications, consequences, and treatment of alcoholism in women, and on the differences between men and women regarding the disposition and effect of alcohol. It is concluded that female alcoholics are a heterogeneous group, and their reasons for drinking can differ not only from men's but also from other women's. A study of 44 alcoholic women found a high prevalence of sexual problems such as rape, incest, orgasmic difficulties, and homosexual experiences. Women have more efficient kidneys than men, which is offset by a tendency to develop higher blood pressure due to hormonal changes at menopause, possibly causing problems in the way their bodies react to unreasonable amounts of alcohol. A relatively larger amount of fatty tissue, with a lower water content to dilute the alcohol, may also put women at a disadvantage. Weight, size, hormone levels, and emotional state are important factors that determine how quickly alcohol affects the brain and other vital organs. A clinical effect of alcohol that is particularly troubling to menopausal women is osteoporosis. The interaction of alcohol and drugs is a special problem for women because they are the prime consumers of prescription medicine. A chapter on helping alcoholics includes a list of major organizations, public and private, that deal with problem drinking. (RUCAS)

494. Levendel, L., Mezei, Á., Nemes, L., & Várady, T. Über die persönlichkeit der alkoholiker und ihre führung in der tuberkulose-heilanstalt. [On the personality of alcoholics and their management in the tuberculosis sanitarium.] *Beiträge zur Klinik der Tuberkulose,* 1964, *128,* 131–145.

The literature on the personality of alcoholics is reviewed. About half showed sexual deviations such as impotence and homosexual tendencies. (NCALI)

495. Mendelson, J. H., & Mello, N. K. Behavioral and biochemical interrelations in alcoholism. *Annual Review of Medicine,* 1976, *27,* 321–333.

A brief review of recent research on the interrelationships between behavioral and biochemical concomitants of alcoholism is presented. The review is focused on 4 specific areas: (1) tolerance and physical dependence, (2) alcohol-induced changes in sexual behavior and function, (3) alcohol-induced liver disease, and (4) the contribution of genetic factors to alcohol problems. Implications of knowledge in these areas for treatment and medical management of the alcoholic individual are noted, and research to fill the remaining gaps in such knowledge is encouraged.

496. Sha'ked, A. *Human sexuality in physical and mental illnesses and disabilities: An annotated bibliography.* Bloomington, IN: Indiana University Press, 1978.

This bibliography encompasses sexual functioning in a variety of disabling conditions. Among these is alcoholism, which is addressed in a chapter devoted to the impact of substance abuse on diverse aspects of human sexuality. The 23 citations in this section all appear in the appropriate chapters of the present volume.

497. U.S. Department of Health, Education, and Welfare. *First special report to the U.S. Congress on alcohol and health.* (DHEW Publication No. HSM 73-9031.) Washington, DC: U.S. Government Printing Office, 1971.

In a brief summary of previous research, it is reported that large doses of alcohol deteriorate sexual performance; alcoholics have disturbed sex lives and show a tendency toward early degeneration of sex glands.

498. Wilson, G. T. Alcohol and human sexual behavior. *Behaviour Research and Therapy,* 1977, *15,* 239–252.

Despite the potential clinical significance of the relationship between alcohol consumption and human sexual responsiveness, the subject has received little systematic research attention. Clinical observations have suggested that alcohol abuse can lead to impotency disorders in males and sexual dysfunction in women. Alcohol has been associated with sex offenses such as rape and pedophilia, increased sexual activity, and extramarital affairs. However, correlation has been confused with cause, and unequivocal evidence of alcohol as the causal agent is lacking. Recent research using penile tumescence and vaginal pressure pulse as measures of sexual arousal has shown a significant negative linear relation between alcohol and sexual responsiveness in both male and female social drinkers. Findings that cognitive rather than pharmacological factors decisively influence alcohol's effects on sexual arousal, together with other psychosocial analyses, dispute the disinhibition hypothesis of alcohol's effects. A social learning analysis of alcohol's influence on sex is proposed. (Author)

B. Psychoanalytic Commentary

499. Abraham, K. [The psychological relations between sexuality and alcoholism.] *International Journal of Psychoanalysis*, 1926, 7, 2–10. (Translated and reprinted from Die psychologischen beziehungen zwischen sexualität und alkoholismus. *Zeitschrift für Sexualwissenschaft*, 1908, 1, 449–458.)

According to this turn-of-the-century paper, male and female sexuality proceed from bisexuality to the aggressive male and passive female. Sexual activity is normally sublimated in both. Alcohol removes the sublimation of sexual energies. Normal repugnancy to perversions is dispelled and taboos are overcome. Male sexual capacity is increased. Female resistance to the male is weakened; therefore, her sexual attraction is weakened. Women who like alcohol are probably homosexual. Chronic drinkers have lost their finer feelings of sublimation. Normal sexual activity is forfeited in the long-term alcoholic. The alcoholic denies his/her alcoholism just as the neurotic denies his/her symptoms, as it is his/her form of sexual activity. The male drinker's jealousy is a manifestation of his displaced guilt over having turned from women to alcohol. Social environment, faulty training, or heredity are not sufficient explanation of alcoholism. Psychoanalysis must be applied, and one must keep in mind the connection between alcoholism and sexuality. (RUCAS)

500. Bergler, E. The psychological interrelation between alcoholism and genital sexuality. *Journal of Criminal Psychology*, 1942, 4, 1–13.

The author argues his objections to commonly held notions on the causes of alcoholism. Theoretical explanations approaching from the side of consciousness amount to taking seriously the patients' rationalizations and do not take into account important unconscious motivations. The psychoanalytic position that alcoholism is the expression of unconscious regression to the oral phase is incomplete. In addition, there is an unconscious wish for revenge for oral denial. For alcoholics, alcohol does not enhance sexuality: it provokes oral revenge fantasies. Sexual behavior and dysfunction are used in defense against these fantasies: (1) they create situations leading to disappointment; (2) alcoholics will hold their spouses responsible for the disappointment and self-righteously attack them; and (3) the end result is the masochistic pleasure of self-pity. Case histories and literary passages illustrate the author's theoretical position. For instance, a female alcoholic when intoxicated would attack her husband with accusations of sexual neglect and lack of love. When her husband attempted intercourse she proved "frigid." (RUCAS)

501. Clark, L. P. A psychological study of some alcoholics. *Psychoanalytic Review*, 1919, 6, 268–295.

One may say that excessive alcoholic indulgence is prompted by unconscious motives. These concern the emotional life and the sexual striving especially. The conscious inadequacy is due to fixations or arrests in emotional development. Alcohol thus liberates in an almost experimental manner the fundamental faults in the psychosexual evolution. That the mental content in alcoholics is so frequently a homosexual one shows the powerful motivation in alcoholics of the special phase of the psychosexual life concerned with sexual identity formation. Many alcoholics illustrate deeper and deeper regressions as they approach profound narcosis—so that one and the same case may show homosexual, narcissistic, and primary maternal identifications as the deeper fixations are brought to the surface. Finally, some agent like alcohol is so universally used because of the common defect and imperfection of our psychosexual life and its improper or inadequate sublimation. Case histories, which present a variety of ways in which alcoholics' sexual lives are disturbed, are provided to illustrate these ideas. (Author)

502. Descombey, J. P. *Is there a Freudian theory of dependence?* Paper presented at the Twenty-seventh International Institute on the Prevention and Treatment of Alcoholism, Vienna, June 1981.

Characteristic features of the Freudian theory of alcohol dependence, alcohol withdrawal symptoms, and drunkenness are explained, and possible directions of development are outlined for a theory based on rigorous clinical experience. (NCALI)

503. Descombey, J. P. La dépendance alcoolique: Problèmes de théorie Freudienne et de technique psychothérapique. [Alcoholic dependence: Problems with Freudian theory and psychotherapeutic technique.] *L'Information Psychiatrique*, 1982, 58, 505–515.

After having recapitulated the elements of Freudian theory on alcohol dependence, the author examines the problems of psychotherapy for clients and psychoanalysts. Inadequacies of the theory and subsequent rationalizations on the part of patients and therapists result in frustration for both. A variety of points of view and therapeutic approach are briefly discussed. The author concludes that, despite the shortcomings of psychoanalysis, therapeutic approaches based on psychoanalytic theory have the best potential for success, for alcoholism has its roots in infantile sexuality.

504. Deutsch, H. Alkohol und homosexualität. [Alcohol and homosexuality.] *Wiener Klinische Wochenschrift*, 1913, *26*, 102–103.

505. Hart, H. H. Personality factors in alcoholism. *Archives of Neurology and Psychiatry*, 1930, *24*, 116–134.

The author argues the position that constitutional deficiencies acquired through heredity, traumatic childhood experiences, and poor training during childhood produce the defective personalities, deceptiveness, and unreliability characteristic of alcoholics. Thirty case histories, 25 male and 5 female alcoholics, are presented to illustrate his position. In a section summarizing sexual adjustment, the author reports a large portion of his sample engaging in irresponsible sexual activity, promiscuity, and infidelity, but little overt homosexuality. The author argues that alcoholics' sexual difficulties and preference for same-sex drinking companions are not due to latent homosexuality as assumed by psychoanalytic theory but rather are due to a constitutional deficiency leaving the alcoholic incapable of adjusting to the responsibilities of adult life.

506. Juliusburger, O. Alkoholismus und psychosexualität. [Alcoholism and psychosexuality.] *Zeitschrift für Sexualwissenschaft*, 1916, *2*, 357–366.

According to the author of this early paper, alcoholism is innate, not produced by environment. Alcoholics have primary need for intoxication. Alcoholism is atavistic like crime. Atavism and a lack of sublimation mechanism are responsible for drinking, not only sexuality. The alcoholic is a defective personality; alcoholism cannot be explained only on the basis of homosexuality. Alcoholism is the equivalent of autoerotic masturbation. The alcoholic is a person with congenital defect, who suffers from constitutionally handicapped development and whose sexual instincts are part of a general developmental retardation. (RUCAS)

507. Karpman, B. *The alcoholic woman: Case studies in the psychodynamics of alcoholism.* Washington, DC: The Linacre Press, 1948.

Case studies of 3 alcoholic women are presented with detailed information on their growing up, the development of their alcoholism, and their adult sexual adjustment. In all 3, alcohol played a role in facilitating sexual behavior. Cases are discussed in the context of psychoanalytic theory, and each represents a different pathway to the development of alcoholism: 1) unconscious, unresolved, incestuous desire for father leading to promiscuity facilitated by alcoholism, 2) childhood maternal deprivation producing intense longing for love expressed in adulthood in paraphiliac behavior usually under the influence of alcohol, 3) conscious homosexuality compelling heterosexual activity accompanied by alcohol abuse to obtain freedom from inhibition, to reduce distaste for men, and to induce forgetfulness of homosexual cravings.

508. Karpman, B. *The Hangover.* Springfield, IL: Charles C. Thomas, 1957.

Fourteen case histories of alcoholic men and women are discussed, focusing on their hangover-related experience. Males' and females' experiences are contrasted. Psychoanalytic interpretations of the alcoholics' behavior and the fantasy material generated during the hangover are offered. The conclusions drawn from these interpretations are that homosexuality and hysteria are the underlying personality pathologies motivating drinking behavior and subsequent hangover experiences.

509. Linczényi, A. Beiträge zur frage der homosexualität. [Contributions to the problem of homosexuality.] *Psychotherapy and Psychosomatics*, 1967, *15*, 40. (Abstract of paper presented at the Seventh International Congress of Psychotherapy, Wiesbaden, 1967.)

A brief case history is presented of a 22-year-old waiter with anxiety and homosexual fantasies, in whom heterosexual stimulation occurred only after alcohol intake. (RUCAS)

510. Näcke, P. Alkohol und homosexualität. [Alcohol and homosexuality.] *Zeitschrift für Psychiatrie*, 1911, *68*, 852–859.

511. Neilsen, N. P., Pra, S. D., Sammarco, A. M., & Veneziani, A. Blacky pictures in the study of personality of chronic alcoholics. *Journal on Alcoholism and Related Addictions*, 1979, *15*, 3–7.

The Blacky Pictures (BP) Test or Blume test is a projective technique modified to psychoanalytical needs that permits the general level of personality development to be controlled. It is designed to locate possible areas of emotional conflict, transposing them to the various phases of psychosexual development. The test consists of 11 tables representing the adventures of a dog named Blacky and a front piece that serves to introduce the characters (Blacky, Father, Mother, and Tippy, the fraternal figure of whom neither age nor sex is specified). The 11 tables represent scenes or situations connected with oral eroticism, oral and anal sadism, Oedipus complex, guilt feeling for masturbation activity, fears of castration, processes of parental identification, fraternal rivalry, guilt feelings, ego ideal, and choice of love object. Results from this test, administered to 32 hospital-based male alcoholic patients in the Provincial Psychiatric Hospital of Como (Italy) and 20 normal subjects, are provided. (NCALI)

512. Neveu, M. P. Homosexualité apparue tardivement sous l'influence d'excès alcooliques. [Homosexuality appearing late in life under the influence of alcohol.] *Annales Medico-Psychologiques*, 1949, *107*, 36–37.

This case history describes a 50-year-old chauffeur who in midlife became obsessed with homosexual fantasies involving adolescent boys. The obsession began following an incident at a party in which the man became intoxicated, lead a 15-year-old boy away from the gathering, then performed anal intercourse. Despite his remorse, he was unable to resist his obsession and made occasional advances toward other boys. The uncharacteristic alcoholic excess in a party setting in the company of a compliant boy released the man's latent homosexuality, resulting in his obsessive preoccupation. This relationship could have been clearly demonstrated with psychoanalysis had psychoanalysis not been contraindicated because of the man's age.

513. Noiville, P. *Alcoolisme, sexualité et dépendance. [Alcoholism, sexuality and dependence.]* Paper presented at 27th International Institute on Prevention and Treatment of Alcoholism, Vienna, June 1981.

The sexuality of a male alcoholic patient as expressed through his phantasmal relations to a woman (heterosexual) or to another man (homosexual) is explained in the framework of structural research of dependence on alcohol. (NCALI)

514. Riggall, R. M. Homosexuality and alcoholism. *Psychoanalytic Review*, 1923, *10*, 157–169.

This is one of the early psychoanalytic essays linking homosexuality with alcoholism. The author attributes homosexuality to faulty psychosexual development, specifically a fixation in infancy on the mother and oral satisfaction. In normal males, latent homosexuality is repressed or sublimated. It is the author's position that alcohol interferes with the sublimation of homosexuality and that alcohol causes regression so that homosexual conflicts are exposed. For example: the affection and camaraderie of men who drink together is seen as an expression of latent homosexuality. In addition, the craving for alcohol is caused, as is homosexuality, by the desire to satisfy unconscious desires for the mother's nipple. Curing alcoholism, therefore, requires correction of psychosexual development through analysis.

515. Salzman, L. Psychodynamics of sexual humor: Sex and alcohol. *Medical Aspects of Human Sexuality*, 1977, *11*, 64–65.

The author provides examples of jokes involving alcohol and sex and offers explanations of these jokes. In all, alcohol allows for greater freedom of expression of sexual interest, reducing prudishness, and enhancing assertiveness or hostility while providing a formidable excuse if it is taken too seriously by the recipient.

516. Sharoff, R. L. Character problems and their relationship to drug abuse. *American Journal of Psychoanalysis*, 1969, *29*, 186–193.

This presentation represents an attempt to characterize the type of individual who is apt to abuse a specific type of drug. Individuals with certain types of problems are more apt to abuse one type of drug than another. The drugs discussed fall into 3 classifications: nonnarcotic sedatives such as alcohol, barbiturates, and minor tranquilizers; narcotics; and hallucinogens, the most common being marijuana, LSD, and mescaline. People who use alcohol or other nonnarcotic sedatives try to resolve character problems related to conflicts dealing with aggression and sex by acting them out. People who use narcotics are trying to resolve problems related to lack of self-esteem. Use of narcotics is a withdrawal from, as well as an attack on, society. People who use hallucinogens have problems related to self-esteem in a competitive, critical society. Drug use enables them to substitute love for competition. Perceptual distortions lead them to feel that they have become in reality what they believe they are in their imaginations.

517. Tausk, V. On the psychology of the alcoholic occupation delirium. *Psychoanalytic Quarterly*, 1969, *38*, 406–431.

This is a psychoanalytic formulation of alcoholic occupation delirium, an alcoholic psychosis in which the delirious patient endlessly performs a routine task. The behavior is compared to the occupation dream, which is a fear of impotence dream. Latent ideas that are demonstrably present in the dream and that lead to changes in occupation correspond to inhibitions that in waking life inhibit the dreamer from obtaining full sexual satisfaction. These patients rarely fail to achieve orgasm, though they rarely achieve psychical satisfaction. Deeper analysis shows a strong homosexual-narcissistic fixation of the libido. More or less pronounced paranoid traits are also found in these cases. The psychical value of their sexual relations is minimal, characterized by the crudest sensuality and lack of erotic or moral respect for the other sex. Alcoholic occupation delirium should be regarded as a coitus-wish delirium strictly analogous to the occupation dream.

C. Miscellaneous Commentary

518. Allen, C. M. Sexuality and substance abuse: Treatment for the troubled family. Seminar 1 (Summary). In D. J. Ottenberg & F. E. Madden (Eds.), *Substance abuse: The family in trouble. Proceedings of the 13th Annual Eagleville Conference, May 1980.* Eagleville, PA: Eagleville Hospital and Rehabilitation Center, 1980.

A summary of a seminar on sexuality and substance abuse is presented, including comments by seminar panelists. (NCALI)

519. Anderson, C. Sexuality and recovery. *The blue book (Vol. 30). Proceedings of the Thirtieth National Clergy Conference on Alcoholism.* New Orleans, January 5–10, 1978. Washington, DC: National Clergy Conference on Alcoholism, 1979.

A Lutheran minister whose pastoral work has been in alcoholism treatment speaks to Catholic clergy and laypersons on sexuality during recovery from alcoholism. Sexuality is conceptualized as a built-in biological drive and is by design intended for relationships. The most important problem observed in the treatment of alcoholism is the area of accepting sexual feelings as normal. Feelings of guilt and self-reproach compound feelings of low self-esteem in the alcoholic. For the religious alcoholic who has chosen a celibate lifestyle unresolved or unrecognized anger over sexual deprivation is exacerbated, especially if abstinence is seen as deprivation as well. Recommendations for pastoral counseling include developing a supportive and safe atmosphere as well as affirming religious faith.

520. Anthony, S. B. *Woman alcoholic: An holistic approach.* Paper presented at the Psychiatric Institute Foundation Conference on Alcoholism, Washington, DC, October 1978.

A holistic approach to female alcoholism is presented as one that recognizes and addresses the interaction between the person and her psychosocial environment (e.g., alcohol intoxication increases vulnerability to rape and creates conditions for sexual encounters which increase exposure to VD and the possibility of unwanted pregnancy). The physical, psychological, social, and economic differences between male and female alcoholism are reviewed, and political and theological aspects of female alcoholism are identified. Holistic healing techniques are described, and their application to prevention and treatment of female alcoholism is recommended. (NCALI)

521. Bell, R. R. Alcohol. In R. R. Bell, *Social deviance: A substantive analysis.* Homewood, IL: Dorsey, 1971.

The literature on alcoholism is reviewed and discussed in the context of alcoholism as social deviance and its impact on social institutions such as the criminal justice system and the family. Within the family, the sexual relationship of the spouses is disturbed by emotional withdrawal on the part of the nonalcoholic partner and by alcohol-induced sexual dysfunction. The tavern or bar is a public meeting place where regular customers may find a sense of community. It serves also as a marketplace for sex—for a fee or free, heterosexual and homosexual.

522. Benjafield, J. G., & Rutter, L. F. Diagnostic tests in alcoholism. *British Journal of Addictions,* 1972, *67,* 231–234.

Alcoholism is gaining increasing recognition as a disease, but etiology is as yet obscure, and symptoms such as excessive drinking and hangovers are unspecific in distinguishing the "true" alcoholic from the less seriously affected heavy drinker. An already difficult situation facing the G.P. or consultant, involving as it does medical, legal, and social implications, threatens to become worse with the possible introduction of compulsory treatment. Data from a 7-year investigation of biochemical and genetic factors in 44 male and 21 female long-recovered and abstinent alcoholics form the basis of a number of tests, some of which are applicable in the surgery, and others within the resources of the normally equipped hospital laboratory. The results, in conjunction with case histories, allow an assessment of alcoholic status which is largely independent of patients' statements, and in doubtful cases assist in deciding whether the patient is "at risk." In males, impotence is common, and some feminization may occur. Incidence of latent or overt homosexuality is high in alcoholics. In women long-standing menstrual irregularities are common. Sexual and psychosexual problems may predispose to alcoholism and therefore warrant attention. (Author)

523. Carver, A. E. The interrelationship of sex and alcohol. *The International Journal of Sexology,* 1948, *11,* 78–81.

This article summarizes the beliefs of medical professionals during the earlier part of this century. Human behavior toward sex and alcohol was seen as reflecting the essentially nonrational nature of the human animal. Both sex and alcohol involve fundamental urges that are subjected to infinitely varied controls. The primitive urges and rational self-control, hedonism, and asceticism are social forces placing people in a state of perpetual flux. Alcohol's ability to release inhibitions and to dull critical senses facilitates seduction. Thus, alcohol and sex become twin indulgences. Homosexuality is so deeply repressed that it requires more alcohol to release inhibition than does heterosexuality. Such a release usually comes as a shock and may be accompanied by amnesia. More repressed sexual wishes such as sadism require more alcohol for expression. Potency, however, is decreased with increased amounts of alcohol intake. Reproductive cells were believed to be unaffected by alcohol. Venereal disease was no more common among drinkers than among abstainers. The consensus was that the worst evil resulting from excessive drinking was in making homelife unsuitable for children. A final observation is that, for some, an alcoholic spree becomes a substitute for orgasm. Alcohol supplants and destroys the activity whose freedom it was introduced to liberate and is a "dangerous medicine for the sexually repressed."

524. Ewing, J. A. How to help the alcoholic marriage. In D. W. Abse, E. M. Nash, & L. M. R. Louden, (Eds.), *Marital and sexual counseling in medical practice.* New York: Harper & Row, 1974.

Alcoholism is discussed in terms of a diversity of underlying disabilities having their roots in personality development and the influence of culture on the development of attitudes toward alcohol. Underlying personality conflicts around sexuality, dependence, and aggression are seen as primary in developing the personality characteristics predisposing an individual to alcoholism. These personality features play an important role in the dynamics of the alcoholic marriage. Guidelines for recognizing alcohol problems and for alcoholism counselling are provided.

525. Ewing, J. A., Fox, R., Carstairs, G. M., & Beaubrun, M. H. Roundtable: Alcohol, drugs, and sex. *Medical Aspects of Human Sexuality,* 1970, *4,* 18–19; 23–25; 28–29; 32–34.

A panel consisting of R. Fox, G. M. Carstairs, and M. H. Beaubrun, moderated by J. A. Ewing, discussed impotence associated with alcohol abuse and the cultural differences in sexual behavior associated with alcohol intoxication. The sexual relationship in marriage is seen as deteriorating along with the marital relationship as drinking increases. One may be repelled by the other's drinking, may cease to enjoy sex, and may try to avoid the sexual relationship. The physiological effects of alcohol may impede the husband's ability to get and maintain an erection and in women render attainment of orgasm more difficult. Use of disulfiram (Antabuse) in the high dosages prescribed in the late 1940s, when disulfiram was first used in the treatment of alcoholism, sometimes led to impotence. The lower dosage used currently presents no such problem. Consideration was given to the psychoanalytic position that latent homosexuality was an etiological factor in both alcoholism and impotence. Evidence, however, does not demonstrate more homosexual behavior among alcoholics. The panelists agree that once drinking has stopped, sexual functioning can return to normal if the mari-

526. Fox, R. Interview: A psychiatrist discusses drinking and sex. *Sexual Behavior,* 1971, *1,* 67–69.

In a question and answer session, the author discusses male and female sexual dysfunction arising from overindulgence in alcohol, the disinhibiting effect of alcohol, and the relationship between homosexuality and alcohol use.

tal relationship has not been too severely damaged. Drinking behavior in Scottish, Caribbean, American, and Asian Indian cultures were compared with regard to the sexual abuses following excesses in alcohol consumption. Venereal disease, prostitution, and unwanted pregnancies are seen as sex-related problems that are associated with alcohol abuse. In general, cultures associate alcohol consumption with sexual prowess. In contrast, use of alcohol in India was associated with sexual inadequacy. A regular user was considered no longer to be a sexual partner.

527. Gebhard, P. H. Situational factors affecting human sexual behavior. In F. A. Beach (Ed.), *Sex and Behavior.* New York: Wiley, 1965.

The interviews and studies conducted by staff members of the Institute for Sex Research bring to awareness the importance of the role played by situational factors in directing human sexual behavior. It is convenient to divide the several situational factors roughly into 3 categories. First are the factors that directly affect the physiological state of the human body with little or no cerebration involved. Second are the cultural factors, the pervasive and powerful influences exerted upon the individual by the society within which he/she lives. Third are the specific, immediate situational factors that exist within, yet are somewhat independent of, the first and second categories. A man's current physiological condition may make him capable and desirous of sexual activity and his cultural environment may encourage him to seek heterosexual satisfaction, but what he actually does is determined by a specific immediate situational factor: the presence or absence of a cooperative female. Most of the information to be presented in the chapter is not in the quantified form. Alcohol and other drugs contribute to the individual's sexual behavior by affecting physiological state. Small to moderate amounts of alcohol or some other drugs may promote sexual activity by lowering inhibitions, causing euphoria, and greasing the wheels of social interaction, but large amounts of the same substances decrease sexuality. Alcoholics and drug addicts frequently engage in little or no sexual activity. The minimal sexuality of alcoholics and addicts may be due in large part to the malnutrition commonly seen in such individuals. (Author)

528. Greaves, G. Towards an existential theory of drug dependence. *The Journal of Nervous and Mental Disease,* 1974, *159,* 263–274.

The author examines 5 leading theories of drug dependence—(a) the acquired drive theory, (b) the avoidance paradigm theory, (c) the metabolic disease theory, (d) the conditioning theory, and (e) the automedication theory—and finds them all lacking. He explores drug dependence within the context of "passive euphoria" and suggests that persons who become drug dependent are those who are not able, for reasons of attitudes or other factors, to create euphoria in usual ways, e.g., engaging in sexual activity. He argues further that most drug programs err seriously by failing to help the drug-dependent person to find euphoric' alternatives to drugs. Because of the ascetic orientation of most drug programs, they thus tend to undermine the very goal for which they strive. (Author)

529. Hammond, D. C., & Jorgensen, G. Q. Alcohol and sex: A volatile cocktail. *USA Today*, July 1981, pp. 44–46.

The following topics are addressed in a discussion of sexuality and alcoholism: (1) erectile dysfunction, (2) testicular damage and failure, (3) hormonal imbalance and feminization, (4) relationship factors in sexual dysfunction, (5) female alcoholism, and (6) fetal alcoholism syndrome. (NCALI)

530. Johnson, J. Havelock Ellis and his "studies in the psychology of sex." *British Journal of Psychiatry*, 1979, *134*, 522–527.

The life of Havelock Ellis is described; his personality and life experiences are related to the writing of his major work. Important sections of the "Studies" are summarized and their relevance to contemporary sexology is emphasized. He continually emphasized Victorian views on alcoholism, its detrimental effects on sexual life and its harmful effects upon the fetus in the intoxicated pregnant woman. He cited experimental evidence from 1906 on the teratogenic effects of alcohol in pregnant animals to support his assertions on its effects in humans. (Author)

531. Miles, W. R. Psychological factors in alcoholism. *Mental Hygiene*, 1937, *21*, 529–548.

The knowledge and thinking about alcoholism during the post-prohibition era are discussed. The impact of prohibition on alcoholism and public attitudes toward prohibition are presented along with supporting statistics. Based on observations of hospitalized alcoholics, the alcoholic's personality is described in terms of immaturity and impulsiveness. Comparisons are made with homosexuals, with the implication of underlying homosexuality in the alcoholic personality. Psychopathic traits are attributed to alcoholics. This is accompanied by statistics comparing temperate, intemperate, and abstinent criminal offenders. Crimes of violence and sexual offenses are attributed to constitutional psychopathic impulsiveness disinhibited by alcohol intoxication. Treatments for alcoholism which were in vogue at the time are discussed.

532. National Clergy Conference on Alcoholism. *The blue book (Vol. 30). Proceedings of the Thirtieth National Clergy Conference on Alcoholism, New Orleans, January 5–10, 1978.* Washington, DC: Author, 1978.

This book represents the proceedings of the Thirtieth National Clergy Conference on Alcoholism and includes 36 presentations on a wide variety of topics related to alcoholism in Catholic priests, nuns, and brothers; included are a bibliography for conference members on topics such as

spiritual aids, counselling, sexuality, self-knowledge, and drugs, a list of recommended treatment facilities, and a directory of participants. (RUCAS)

533. National Institute on Alcohol Abuse and Alcoholism. *Alcoholism and alcohol abuse among women: Research issues. Proceedings of a workshop, Jekyll Island, Georgia, April 1978.* (NIAAA Research Monograph No. 1, DHEW Publication No. ADM-80-835.) Washington, DC: U.S. Government Printing Office, 1980.

This document contains the 6 lectures, the discussion summaries, and the recommendations of a workshop on alcoholism in women. The lectures describe drinking surveys, biological and psychosocial consequences of alcohol problems among women (including physiological and psychological vulnerability), clinical, education, and prevention aspects. (RUCAS)

534. Ottenberg, D. J., & Madden, E. E. (Eds.). *Substance abuse: The family in trouble. Proceedings of the 13th Annual Eagleville Conference, Eagleville, PA, May 1980.* Eagleville, PA: Eagleville Hospital and Rehabilitation Center, 1980.

Papers, seminars, and training modules presented at the Thirteenth Annual Eagleville Conference are provided. Topics addressed in these papers include program sensitivity to minority services, medical perspectives of substance abuse and the family, a family theory of drug abuse, and substance abuse and the family. The seminars and training modules focus on the following topics: (1) sexuality and substance abuse (treatment for the troubled family), (2) violence and substance abuse, (3) disintegration through substance abuse (family in pain), (4) the older adult and substance abuse (alcohol, medication, and the aging process), (5) ethnic minorities and the economically disadvantaged (identifying problems and finding solutions in the delivery of service), and (6) the young and substance abuse (approaching multi-problem youth and their families). A brief historical background on the development of the Eagleville Hospital and Rehabilitation Center (Pennsylvania), and the Thirteenth Annual Donovan Lecture, "Myth and Reality in the Family Patterns and Treatment of Substance Abusers," are also presented. (NCLAI)

535. Paret, R. L., Carrasco, J. S-D., & Catalan, R. C. Coloquio: Sexualidad y alcoholismo. [Colloquium: Sexuality and alcoholism.] *Sexualmedica*, 1974, *8*, 69–72.

536. Pierce, B. Mental states in alcoholism. *The Lancet*, 1924, *1*, 841–843.

Some clinical varieties of mental disorder are due to alcohol intemperance: alcoholic delirium (delirium tremens), transient mania (mania a potu), acute alcohol hallucinosis, and polyneuritic psychosis (Korsakov's Syndrome). The primitive instincts, the herd instinct, the sexual instinct, and the ego instinct, are markedly affected by alcoholism. The sexual instinct becomes less under control resulting in crimes of passion and indecencies of all kinds.

537. Sherfey, M. J. Psychopathology and character structure in chronic alcoholism. In O. Diethelm (Ed.), *Etiology of chronic alcoholism.* Springfield, IL: Thomas, 1955.

On the basis of this study of the underlying psychopathology and personalities of 161 cases of chronic alcoholism, the author concludes that alcoholism is a symptom associated with several illnesses or syndromes. An adequate differential diagnosis is necessary for the understanding of each case. Subjects in some diagnostic categories exhibited characteristic sexual adjustment behaviors. The cases with well-defined diagnostic categories are: (a) paranoid schizophrenia (14 cases)—latent homosexual features and delusions and hallucinations of homosexual content are more evident here than in any other group; (b) manic-depressive reactions (11 cases)—onset of illness and excessive drinking coincided in all cases, depressions were light, agitated depressions were complicated by the intoxication and tended to be associated with premenstrual or postpartum intervals in the women; (c) poorly organized, asocial psychopathic personalities (11 male cases)—sexual behavior was rarely attempted when sober, the subjects exhibited an inability to form a satisfying sexual relationship with women, promiscuity, impotence, and homosexuality were prominent; (d) poorly organized, psychoneurotic psychopathic personality (15 cases, only females)—subjects' chaotic sexuality included frigidity, masturbation, promiscuity, and all forms of perversion as well as some obvious homosexual conflict; and (e) brain damage (5 cases)—onset of alcohol abuse associated with personality change (one case developed exhibitionistic sexual behavior). Some cases did not belong to any usual diagnostic category: (a) rigidly organized, obsessive-compulsive personality (22 cases, all relatively successful middle-aged, 41–60-yr-old males)—subjects exhibited poor heterosexual adjustment, were rarely promiscuous except when intoxicated, commonly suffered premature ejaculation, impotence, and fear of impotence and, though it was not frequently apparent, when latent homosexuality did occur it was accompanied by paranoid projections; (b) rigidly organized neurotic personalities with paranoid features (17 female cases)—subjects exhibited masculine identifications and pervasive psychosexual conflict, some homosexuality, frequently frigidity or strong unsatisfied sexual tension, and their alcoholism began with marriage or with their attempt at heterosexual adjustment, resulting in early intoxications, their ignoring their husbands and being erotic with other men or women, later becoming belligerent, cruel, suspicious and promiscuous; (c) poorly organized, inadequate personality (30 male cases)—subjects were passive with strong dependency needs and fear of responsibility, suffered impotence, fear of impotence, and in one case only, homosexuality; (d) dependent psychoneurotic personalities with depression and tension (12 female cases)—subjects exhibited some frigidity, rarely promiscuity, (e) middle and late life depression (5 male, 6 female)—subjects were quiet while sober but became dishevelled and obscene when intoxicated, resulting in sexual exposure and public scenes.

538. Springer, A., Burian, W., Demel, I., Köhler, I., & Mader, R. Suchtverhalten und geschlechtlichkeit.

[Addictive behavior and sexuality.] *Suchtgefahren,* 1978, *24,* 121–123.

539. Todd, W. H. The truth about sex and alcohol. *Memorial Mercury,* 1973, *13,* 15–16.

Alcohol may be a mild aphrodisiac, but more likely it removes inhibitions. In the middle-aged person, sexual performance is affected very soon after ingestion, thus impairment of performance is almost immediate. Resulting failure may lead to serious anxiety over the possibilities of permanent failure, loss of libido, and eventually psychological impotence. It is speculated that many broken marriages are the result of this chain of events induced by alcohol. Sexual functioning is even more dramatically affected in the later stages of alcoholism. Cirrhosis of the liver in the male makes the elimination of female hormones impossible, resulting in a build-up of large amounts of female hormones. This build-up causes breast enlargement, loss of muscle, loss of body hair, and atrophy of the testicles. Impotence is inevitable. (NCALI)

540. Walton, A. H. Drink, tobacco, crime and sex. *Journal of Sex Education,* 1951, *3,* 128–131.

Overindulgence in alcohol, tobacco, gambling, and petty crime are seen as indicative of sexual neurosis. Substances and behaviors, when indulged to excess, are substitutes for repressed and inhibited sexual expression. When wholesome attitudes toward sexuality exist, the need for substitute behaviors is removed.

541. Winick, C. Substances of abuse and sexual behavior. In J. H. Lowinson & P. Ruiz (Eds.), *Substance abuse: Clinical problems and perspectives.* Baltimore, MD: Williams & Wilkins, 1981.

In this chapter, an overview of current knowledge on sexuality and substances of abuse (aphrodisiacs, opiates, barbiturates, tranquilizers, LSD, cocaine, amphetamine, amyl nitrate, marijuana, and alcohol), in terms of substance effects on sex, is presented. The association of alcohol, sexual problems, and violence is discussed, including sexual problems in the treatment of the alcoholic. (NCALI)

542. Zuckerman, M. Experience: Sex, drugs, alcohol, smoking, and eating. In M. Zuckerman, *Sensation seeking: Beyond the optimal level of arousal.* (Vol. 14). Hillsdale, NJ: Lawrence Erlbaum, 1979.

The thesis is presented that activities involving sex, drugs, alcohol, smoking, and eating are sources of sensory stimulation and arousal; and studies linking sensation seeking with the use of drugs and alcohol are discussed. In student and nonstudent populations, persons who experiment with a variety of drugs tend to be high sensation seekers relative to alcohol users and total abstainers. There tends to be a correlation between number of drugs tried and sensation seeking, except in younger college populations, where many drug users are just beginning to experiment with milder drugs (marijuana and hashish). Alcohol use tends to be associated with a more narrow kind of sensation seeking, that of the "disinhibition" type in college populations and "boredom susceptibility" in veterans' populations. Older alcoholics appear to be average for their age on all sensation-seeking scales. (RUCAS)

V. Appendices

A. Resources for Alcohol Information

1. Al-Anon Family Group, Inc.
   P.O. Box 182
   Madison Square Station
   New York, NY 10159

2. Alcoholics Anonymous World Services, Inc.
   Box 459
   Grand Central Station
   New York, NY 10163

3. Alcoholics Together (AT) Center
   3596 Beverly Boulevard
   Los Angeles, CA 90004

4. Center of Alcohol Studies*
   Information Services Division
   Rutgers University
   P.O. Box 969
   Piscataway, NJ 08854

5. Do It Now Foundation
   P.O. Box 5115
   Phoenix, AZ 85010

6. National Association for Gay Alcoholism Professionals (NAGAP)
   P.O. Box 376
   Oakland, NJ 07436

7. National Clearinghouse for Alcohol Information (NCALI)*
   U.S. Department of Health & Human Services
   National Institute on Alcohol Abuse and Alcoholism
   P.O. Box 2345
   Rockville, MD 20852

8. National Council on Alcoholism (NCA)
   Public Information Department
   733 Third Avenue
   New York, NY 10017

9. Wisconsin Clearinghouse
   University of Wisconsin Hospital and Clinic
   1954 East Washington Avenue
   Madison, WI 53704

*Note: These resource centers include a computerized database of the alcoholism literature and provide literature searches as a service.

B. Resources for Information on Sexuality

1. American Association of Sex Educators, Counselors and Therapists (AASECT)
   5010 Wisconsin Avenue, N.W.
   Washington, DC 20016

2. Kinsey Institute for Sex Research*
   Information Service
   416 Morrison Hall
   Indiana University
   Bloomington, IN 47405

3. Masters & Johnson Institute
   4910 Forest Park Boulevard
   St. Louis, MO 63108

4. Sex Information and Education Council of the U.S. (SIECUS)
   SIECUS Resource Center & Library
   51 West Fourth Street, Room 53
   New York University
   New York, NY 10003

*Note: This resource center includes a computerized database of the sexuality literature and provides literature searches as a service.

C. Representative Sexuality Journals

1. *Archives of Sexual Behavior*
   Plenum Publishing Corporation
   227 West 17 Street
   New York, NY 10011

2. *Journal of Homosexuality*
   Haworth Press
   149 Fifth Avenue
   New York, NY 10010

3. *Journal of Sex & Marital Therapy*
   Behavioral Publications, Inc.
   72 Fifth Avenue
   New York, NY 10011

4. *Journal of Sex Education and Therapy*
   American Association of Sex Educators and
   Counselors
   5010 Wisconsin Avenue
   Washington, DC 20016

5. *Journal of Sex Research*
   The Society for the Scientific Study of Sex, Inc.
   12 East 41st Street
   New York, NY 10017

6. *Medical Aspects of Human Sexuality*
   Hospital Publications, Inc.
   609 Fifth Avenue
   New York, NY 10011

7. *Sexology*
   SXO Corporation
   200 Park Avenue South
   New York, NY 10003

8. *Sexual Behavior*
   Interpersonal Publications, Inc.
   299 Park Avenue
   New York, NY 10017

9. *Sexual Medicine Today*
   600 New Hampshire Avenue, N.W.
   Washington, DC 20037

10. *Sexuality and Disability*
    Human Sciences Press
    72 Fifth Avenue
    New York, NY 10011

11. *SIECUS Report*
    Sex Information and Education Council of the U.S.
    Publications Office
    1855 Broadway
    New York, NY 10023

D. Representative Alcohol Journals

1. *Addictive Behaviors: An International Journal*
   Peter M. Miller, Editor
   Department of Behavioral Medicine
   Hilton Head Hospital
   P.O. Box 1117
   Hilton Head Island, SC 29928

2. *Addictive Diseases: An International Journal*
   Spectrum Publications
   86-19 Sancho Street
   Holliswood, NY 11423

3. *Advances in Alcohol and Substance Abuse*
   Haworth Press
   149 Fifth Avenue
   New York, NY 10010

4. *Alcohol Health and Research World*
   National Institute on Alcohol Abuse and
   Alcoholism
   Box 2345
   Rockville, MD 20852

5. *Alcoholism: Clinical and Experimental Research*
   National Council on Alcoholism
   733 Third Avenue
   New York, NY 10017

6. *Alcoholism & Drug Addiction Research Foundation Journal*
   Addiction Research Foundation of Ontario
   33 Russell Street
   Toronto, Ontario M5S 2S1
   Canada

7. *American Journal of Drug & Alcohol Use*
   Marcel Dekker Journals
   P.O. Box 11305
   Church Street Station
   New York, NY 10249

8. *British Journal of Addiction*
   Society for the Study of Addiction to Alcohol and
   Other Drugs
   Longman Group Ltd., Journals Division
   43–45 Annandale Street
   Edinburgh EH7 4AT, Scotland

9. *British Journal of Alcohol & Alcoholism*
   Medical Council on Alcoholism
   B. Edsall & Co. Ltd.
   36 Eccleston Square
   London, S.W.1., England

10. *Contemporary Drug Problems*
    Federal Legal Publications, Inc.
    157 Chambers
    New York, NY 10007

11. *Drug and Alcohol Dependence*
    Elsevier Sequoia SA
    P.O. Box 851
    1001 Lausanne 1, Switzerland

12. *International Journal of the Addictions*
    Marcel Dekker Journals
    P.O. Box 11305
    Church Street Station
    New York, NY 10249

13. *Journal of Drug Education*
    Baywood Publishing Co.
    120 Marine Street
    Farmingdale, NY 11735

14. *Journal of Drug Issues*
    P.O. Box 4021
    Tallahassee, FL 32303

15. *Journal of Studies on Alcohol*
    Center of Alcohol Studies
    Rutgers University
    P.O. Box 969
    Piscataway, NJ 08854

Author Index